Parasomnias

Guest Editor

MARK R. PRESSMAN, PhD, D.ABSM

SLEEP MEDICINE CLINICS

www.sleep.theclinics.com

December 2011 • Volume 6 • Number 4

SAUNDERS an imprint of ELSEVIER, Inc.

W.B. SAUNDERS COMPANY
A Division of Elsevier Inc.

1600 John F. Kennedy Boulevard • Suite 1800 • Philadelphia, PA 19103-2899

http://www.sleep.theclinics.com

SLEEP MEDICINE CLINICS Volume 6, Number 4
December 2011, ISSN 1556-407X, ISBN-13: 978-1-4557-7992-5

Editor: Sarah E. Barth
Developmental Editor: Donald E. Mumford

Sleep Medicine Clinics (ISSN 1556-407X) is published quarterly by Elsevier Inc., 360 Park Avenue South, New York, NY 10010-1710. Months of issue are March, June, September and December. Business and Editorial Offices: 1600 John F. Kennedy Blvd., Ste. 1800, Philadelphia, PA 19103-2899. Customer Service Office: 3251 Riverport Lane, Maryland Heights, MO 63043. Periodicals postage paid at New York, NY and additional mailing offices. Subscription prices are $161.00 per year (US individuals), $80.00 (US residents), $346.00 (US institutions), $198.00 (foreign individuals), $111.00 (foreign residents), and $381.00 (foreign institutions). Foreign air speed delivery is included in all *Clinics* subscription prices. All prices are subject to change without notice. **POSTMASTER:** Send change of address to *Sleep Medicine Clinics*, Elsevier Health Sciences Division, Subscription Customer Service, 3251 Riverport Lane, Maryland Heights, MO 63043. Customer Service: **Tel: 1-800-654-2452 (U.S. and Canada); 314-447-8871 (outside U.S. and Canada). Fax: 314-447-8029. E-mail: journalscustomerservice-usa@elsevier.com (for print support); journalsonlinesupport-usa@elsevier.com (for online support).**

Reprints. For copies of 100 or more of articles in this publication, please contact the Commercial Reprints Department, Elsevier Inc., 360 Park Avenue South, New York, NY 10010-1710. Tel.: 212-633-3812; Fax: 212-462-1935; E-mail: reprints@elsevier.com.

Printed and bound by CPI Group (UK) Ltd, Croydon, CR0 4YY

Transferred to Digital Print 2011

GOAL STATEMENT

The goal of *Sleep Clinics of North America* is to keep practicing physicians up to date with current clinical practice by providing timely articles reviewing the state of the art in patient care.

ACCREDITATION

The *Sleep Clinics of North America* is planned and implemented in accordance with the Essential Areas and Policies of the Accreditation Council for Continuing Medical Education (ACCME) through the joint sponsorship of the University of Virginia School of Medicine and Elsevier. The University of Virginia School of Medicine is accredited by the ACCME to provide continuing medical education for physicians.

The University of Virginia School of Medicine designates this enduring material activity for a maximum of 15 *AMA PRA Category 1 Credit*(s)™ for each issue, 60 credits per year. Physicians should only claim credit commensurate with the extent of their participation in the activity.

The American Medical Association has determined that physicians not licensed in the US who participate in this CME enduring material activity are eligible for a maximum of 15 *AMA PRA Category 1* Credit(s)™ for each issue, 60 credits per year.

Credit can be earned by reading the text material, taking the CME examination online at http://www.theclinics.com/home/cme, and completing the evaluation. After taking the test, you will be required to review any and all incorrect answers. Following completion of the test and evaluation, your credit will be awarded and you may print your certificate.

FACULTY DISCLOSURE/CONFLICT OF INTEREST

The University of Virginia School of Medicine, as an ACCME accredited provider, endorses and strives to comply with the Accreditation Council for Continuing Medical Education (ACCME) Standards of Commercial Support, Commonwealth of Virginia statutes, University of Virginia policies and procedures, and associated federal and private regulations and guidelines on the need for disclosure and monitoring of proprietary and financial interests that may affect the scientific integrity and balance of content delivered in continuing medical education activities under our auspices.

The University of Virginia School of Medicine requires that all CME activities accredited through this institution be developed independently and be scientifically rigorous, balanced and objective in the presentation/discussion of its content, theories and practices.

All authors/editors participating in an accredited CME activity are expected to disclose to the readers relevant financial relationships with commercial entities occurring within the past 12 months (such as grants or research support, employee, consultant, stock holder, member of speakers bureau, etc.). The University of Virginia School of Medicine will employ appropriate mechanisms to resolve potential conflicts of interest to maintain the standards of fair and balanced education to the reader. Questions about specific strategies can be directed to the Office of Continuing Medical Education, University of Virginia School of Medicine, Charlottesville, Virginia.

The faculty and staff of the University of Virginia Office of Continuing Medical Education have no financial affiliations to disclose.

The authors/editors listed below have identified no professional or financial affiliations for themselves or their spouse/ partner:
Sarah Barth (Acquisitions Editor); Cynthia Brown, MD (Test Author); Peter R. Buchanan, MD, FRACP; Elena del Busto, MD; A. Roger Ekirch, PhD; Mark W. Mahowald, MD; Angus Nisbet, BMedSci, BM, BS, FRCP; Mathieu Pilon, PhD; Mark R. Pressman, PhD, D.ABSM (Guest Editor); Carlos H. Schenck, MD; John M. Shneerson, MA, DM, MD, FRCP; Naoka Tachibana, MD, PhD; Kenneth J. Weiss, MD; and Antonio Zadra, PhD.

The authors/editors listed below identified the following professional or financial affiliations for themselves or their spouse/partner:
Dev Banerjee, MBChB, MD, FRCP is an industry funded research/investigator for Philips Respironics and Merck, and is on the Advisory Committee/Board for UCB PHarma (UK).
Michel A. Cramer Bornemann, MD receives industry funded research support from Vanda Pharmaceuticals, Pfizer, Inc., Inspire Medical systems, and GSK.
Michael J. Howell, MD receives salary support from Apnex Medical.
Teofilo Lee- Chiong, Jr, MD (Consulting Editor) is an industry funded research/investigator for Respironics and Embla.

Disclosure of Discussion of Non-FDA Approved Uses for Pharmaceutical Products and/or Medical Devices
The University of Virginia School of Medicine, as an ACCME provider, requires that all faculty presenters identify and disclose any off-label uses for pharmaceutical and medical device products. The University of Virginia School of Medicine recommends that each physician fully review all the available data on new products or procedures prior to clinical use.

TO ENROLL

To enroll in the Sleep Clinics of North America Continuing Medical Education program, call customer service at 1-800-654-2452 or visit us online at www.theclinics.com/home/cme. The CME program is available to subscribers for an additional fee of $114.00.

Sleep Medicine Clinics

THE CLINICS ARE NOW AVAILABLE ONLINE!

Access your subscription at:
www.theclinics.com

Contributors

CONSULTING EDITOR

TEOFILO LEE-CHIONG Jr, MD
Professor of Medicine and Chief, Division
of Sleep Medicine, National Jewish Health;
Associate Professor of Medicine, University
of Colorado Denver School of Medicine,
Denver, Colorado

GUEST EDITOR

MARK R. PRESSMAN, PhD, D.ABSM
Director, Sleep Medicine Services, Lankenau
Medical Center and Lankenau Institute for
Medical Research, Wynnewood; Clinical
Professor of Medicine, Department of
Medicine, Jefferson Medical College,
Philadelphia; Adjunct Professor, Villanova
School of Law, Villanova, Pennsylvania

AUTHORS

DEV BANERJEE, MBChB, MD, FRCP
Academic Department of Sleep and
Ventilation, Birmingham Heartlands Hospital,
Heart of England NHS Foundation Trust,
Bordesley Green East; Aston Brain Centre,
School of Life and Health Sciences,
Aston University, Birmingham,
United Kingdom

PETER R. BUCHANAN, MD, FRACP
Senior Clinical Research Fellow, Sleep
and Circadian Research Group, NHMRC
Centre for Integrated Research and
Understanding of Sleep (CIRUS), Woolcock
Institute of Medical Research; Senior Staff
Specialist, Department of Respiratory
Medicine, Liverpool Hospital, Liverpool;
Consultant Sleep Medicine Physician,
Sleep Disorders Service, St Vincent's
Clinic, Darlinghurst, Sydney,
New South Wales, Australia

MICHEL A. CRAMER BORNEMANN, MD
Department of Neurology, Minnesota Regional
Sleep Disorders Center, Hennepin County
Medical Center; and Department of Neurology,
University of Minnesota Medical School,
Minneapolis, Minnesota

ELENA DEL BUSTO, MD
Fellow in Forensic Psychiatry, Department
of Psychiatry, Perelman School of Medicine
at the University of Pennsylvania, Philadelphia,
Pennsylvania

A. ROGER EKIRCH, PhD
Professor of History, Department of History,
Virginia Tech, Blacksburg, Virginia

MICHAEL J. HOWELL, MD
Assistant Professor, Department of Neurology,
University of Minnesota; Director, Parasomnia
Program, University of Minnesota Medical
Center, Minneapolis, Minnesota

MARK W. MAHOWALD, MD
Department of Neurology, Minnesota
Regional Sleep Disorders Center,
Hennepin County Medical Center; and
Department of Neurology, University
of Minnesota Medical School,
Minneapolis, Minnesota

**ANGUS NISBET, BMedSci, BM,
BS, FRCP**
East Grinstead Sleep Disorders
Centre, Queen Victoria Hospital
NHS Foundation Trust, West Sussex,
United Kingdom

MATHIEU PILON, PhD
Center for Advanced Research in Sleep
Medicine, Hôpital du Sacré-Cœur;
Ste-Justine Hospital Research Center,
Montréal, Québec, Canada

MARK R. PRESSMAN, PhD, D.ABSM
Director, Sleep Medicine Services,
Lankenau Medical Center and Lankenau
Institute for Medical Research, Wynnewood;
Clinical Professor of Medicine, Department
of Medicine, Jefferson Medical College,
Philadelphia; Adjunct Professor,
Villanova School of Law, Villanova,
Pennsylvania

CARLOS H. SCHENCK, MD
Department of Psychiatry, Minnesota Regional
Sleep Disorders Center, Hennepin County
Medical Center; and Department of Psychiatry,
University of Minnesota Medical School,
Minneapolis, Minnesota

**JOHN M. SHNEERSON, MA, DM, MD,
FRCP, FCCP**
Director, Respiratory Support and Sleep
Centre, Papworth Hospital, Papworth Everard,
Cambridge, United Kingdom

NAOKO TACHIBANA, MD, PhD
Center for Sleep-Related Disorders, Kansai
Electric Power Hospital, Fukushima, Osaka;
Clinical Professor of Neurology, Tokushima
University Graduate School of Medicine,
Tokushima, Japan

KENNETH J. WEISS, MD
Clinical Associate Professor of Psychiatry,
Department of Psychiatry; Associate Director,
Forensic Psychiatry Fellowship Program,
Perelman School of Medicine at the University
of Pennsylvania, Philadelphia, Pennsylvania

ANTONIO ZADRA, PhD
Professor, Department of Psychology,
Université de Montréal; Center for Advanced
Research in Sleep Medicine, Hôpital du
Sacré-Cœur, Montréal, Québec, Canada

Contents

nocturnal fast can result in adverse health consequences such as inadequate sleep maintenance, weight gain, the consumption of inedible substances, or sleep-related injury. The dysfunctional eating may occur in the setting of sedative-hypnotic medications, in particular the widely prescribed benzodiazepine receptor agonists such as zolpidem, frequently inducing amnesia. SRED is often associated with other sleep disorders, in particular restless legs syndrome, and may be a nonmotor manifestation of this condition.

Impaired driving associated with sedative/hypnotic use is often called sleep driving. Sleep driving is most often described as a variant of sleepwalking. A recent case provides the first complete clinical history and description of a sleep-driving case associated with sleepwalking from beginning to end. Sleepwalking-related behavior accounted for the onset and beginning of the episode. However, residual drug effects were also required to account for the driver's behavior at the end of the episode. Sleepwalking and residual drug effects after an awakening may overlap and be required to account for the impaired driver's behavior.

Sleepwalking (somnambulism) and sleep terrors are known as disorders of arousal, share many characteristics, and constitute 2 of the most frequent and impressive non–rapid eye movement (NREM) sleep parasomnias. This article presents key considerations in the assessment and diagnosis of NREM arousal parasomnias. The use of sleep deprivation before polysomnographic investigations can help capture episodes in the sleep laboratory. Auditory-based forced arousals from patients' slow wave sleep may also induce episodes. These and other investigative tools, including brain imaging, may pave the way toward a better understanding of disorders of arousal.

Rapid eye movement (REM) sleep behavior disorder (RBD) is characterized by dream-enacted behaviors with potential risk for injury to the patient and the bed partner. RBD is classified as a parasomnia in the International Classification of Sleep Disorders. RBD has attracted the attention of sleep researchers and clinicians for three reasons. First, it provides insight about the mechanism of REM-sleep generation. Second, it affects quality of life with social embarrassment, psychological conflict, and possibility of injuries. Third, most RBD is associated with various neurologic disorders, especially with neurodegenerative synucleinopathic diseases, including Parkinson disease, dementia with Lewy bodies, and multiple-system atrophy.

Motor acts during sleep (especially violence) have been a source of mystery and confusion. Before there was a scientific approach to sleep physiology, the jurisprudence of sleep violence was based on clinical descriptions and folk wisdom.

Somnambulism and sleep-drunkenness were often valid excuses for homicidal behavior. Forensic psychiatrist Isaac Ray and legal scholar Francis Wharton were among those who gave serious consideration to the jurisprudence of sleep violence. The celebrated 1846 Boston murder trial of Albert Tirrell shows the way in which the existence of somnambulism was used to excuse homicidal behavior.

Foreword

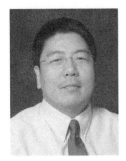

Teofilo Lee-Chiong Jr, MD
Consulting Editor

A man killed his wife by stabbing her twenty-five times with a kitchen knife. A man shot his wife to death with a handgun. A man brutally beat his mother-in-law to death with a tire iron. A mother threw her infant out of a window. A mother killed her daughter with an axe. A father smashed his infant son's head on the floor. A grandfather video-taped his nude five-year-old granddaughter. A man pushed his wife into the family pool and held her head under water until she died. A man got into bed with a seven-year-old girl and tried to pull off her underwear. All these reports allegedly involved violent or abnormal behaviors occurring during the sleep period.

Forensics is increasingly becoming an important aspect of clinical sleep medicine and sleep science research. In its broadest sense, forensic sleep medicine seeks to answer several fundamental questions. What is the prevalence of violent sleep-related activities? How do we deal with the offender? How do we protect potential victims? How do we distinguish sleep-related violent behavior from other violent activities (eg, innate, learned, or defensive)? How should abnormal sleep-related behavior be evaluated? What is the best immediate therapy? What is the best long-term therapy? How effective are these therapies? What type of follow-up is needed? What is the likelihood of recurrence of sleep-related violence? What is the best way to deal with its associated legal issues?

The prevalence of sleep-related violence is unknown, but is considered to be not uncommon. Several sleep disorders are associated with sleep-related violence, including sundowning, confusional arousals, REM sleep behavior disorder, sleep terrors, sleepwalking, and sleep-related seizures. In addition, medication and substance use or abuse can give rise to nocturnal violent activities that can, in certain instances, lead to injuries to the sleeping person, others, or both. Many conditions may act as potential triggers for sleep-related violence, such as stress, sleep deprivation, or disturbances in sleep-wake schedules. Last, the differential diagnosis of sleep-related violence is extensive (eg, dissociative states, alcohol intoxication, fugue, encephalopathy, malingering, Munchausen's by proxy, and, of course, intentional homicide). Thus, it is imperative to define its precise diagnosis, all predisposing factors, and possible mimics.

A comprehensive evaluation is crucial and should involve a thorough accounting of the specific details of the event(s) (ie, time and place of the occurrence, behavior and psychological state of the aggressor, prior violence by the aggressor, and degree of planning needed to perform the act). Sleep, neurological, and psychiatric testing may provide important diagnostic clues. Nonetheless, in many instances, reliable information is unavailable to provide guidance in the determination of criminal intent (if present), and culpability or legal responsibility (if any).

Teofilo Lee-Chiong Jr, MD
Division of Sleep Medicine
National Jewish Health
University of Colorado Denver School of Medicine
1400 Jackson Street, Room J221
Denver, CO 60206, USA

E-mail address:
Lee-ChiongT@NJC.ORG

Sleep Med Clin 6 (2011) xi
doi:10.1016/j.jsmc.2011.08.010
1556-407X/11/$ – see front matter © 2011 Elsevier Inc. All rights reserved.

sleep.theclinics.com

Preface
Common Misconceptions About Sleepwalking and Other Parasomnias

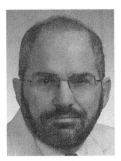

Mark R. Pressman, PhD, D.ABSM
Guest Editor

Parasomnias are behaviors—sometimes complex behaviors—that come out of sleep or out of the transition between sleep and wakefulness.[1] Parasomnias are actually statistically common, but frequently misunderstood by the lay public and those in the medical field.[2] A web search for the term "sleepwalking" brings back hundreds of hits, but rarely for the medical condition. Losing sports teams, governments, and countries are all said to be "sleepwalking." Sleepwalking is used in the sense they are unaware of what is going on around them, not paying attention to what is obvious to others, or moving without purpose or intention. The scientific definition of sleepwalking shares very little with this common understanding. It skims the surface of what we have come to understand is a group of complex and fascinating sleep disorders.

It has been known for hundreds of years that individuals may arouse and/or arise during sleep and perform complex behaviors without conscious awareness or memory of their actions. Early theories of sleepwalking and what we now understand are other types of parasomnias were attributed to demonic or divine possession and other supernatural explanations. Later theories assumed sleepwalkers to be insane or mentally ill. In the 19th century theories evolved with sleepwalking being classified as a sleep disease. Later theories assumed that sleepwalkers must be acting out their dreams. This all occurred before the discovery of

rapid eye movement (REM) sleep in 1953[3] and its later high correlation with dream mentation. Until 1965 sleepwalking was thought to be related to dream enactment and the content of the dreams related to prior psychological traumas. In 1965 the first studies of sleepwalking in a modern sleep laboratory were published.[4,5] Researchers were surprised to find sleepwalking did not occur during REM sleep, but rather during deep non-rapid eye movement (NREM) sleep. An understanding developed that sleepwalking occurred following a partial arousal from deep sleep and was not associated with dreams or dream enactment. The association with partial arousals led Broughton to coin the phrase "Disorders of Arousal" for sleepwalking and related disorders, confusional arousal, and night terrors.[6] Although sleepwalking was often found to be associated with situational stress, sleepwalkers were not found to suffer from underlying psychopathology or mental illness. Research into the diagnosis of sleepwalking and other parasomnias has continued rapidly, especially in the last 10 years. Banerjee and Nisbett in their article in this volume provide an update on issues that affect the clinical diagnosis and treatment of NREM parasomnias.

The concept of sleepwalking has been expanded to include complex sleep-related behaviors other than just walking. These complex behaviors often reflect basic functions of the primitive brain. They include sleep eating, sleep sex, and sleep violence

Sleep Med Clin 6 (2011) xiii–xvii
doi:10.1016/j.jsmc.2011.08.008

(see Howell, and Buchanan, in this volume for detailed information on sleep eating and sleep sex). All are considered variants of sleepwalking as they come out of NREM sleep. Other behaviors are considered "automatic," suggesting they could be performed with little conscious awareness.

Current theories of sleepwalking point to differences in the functional organization of the brain during deep sleep. The sleepwalker's brain appears to be different in the manner in which it handles incoming sensory stimuli. Additional theories suggest local areas in the brain may "sleep" while other areas are active. These neurophysiologic differences point out that many behaviors and disorders are the result of dissociations in the brain between different states of consciousness. Behaviors may be a combination of not just wake and sleep, but wake, REM sleep, and NREM sleep. Mahowald and colleagues review the science of brain state dissociations, sleep and parasomnias in their article in this volume.

In the absence of conscious awareness, sleepwalkers were thought not to be responsible for their behaviors even if those behaviors might be otherwise thought of as criminal. Criminal behavior requires the intent to commit the crime. In the absence of conscious awareness, sleepwalkers were most often not held responsible for their actions. This became especially common in the 19th century when trials employed this defense, although legal cases can be identified more than 500 years ago. The basic defense remains the same today, even though in the 19th century the most important aspects of sleep science, parasomnias, and forensic sleep medicine that we have access to today were of course unknown. Forensic sleep science continues to build on these 19th century criminal cases. This volume contains several articles that review 19th century approaches to sleepwalking and criminal behavior (see Weiss and del Busto, Ekirch and Shneerson, and Shneerson and Ekirch).

In 1985 a new disorder that corresponded to the now disproved concept of sleepwalking as a disorder of dream enactment was discovered.[7] Labeled REM Sleep Behavior Disorder (RBD), it occurred primarily in older men who often went on to develop serious degenerative brain disorders. Current research suggests signs and symptoms of RBD may be a prodromal symptom for synucleinopathies such Parkinson's disease, multiple system atropy, and dementia with Lewy bodies. However, most patients with RBD present to the sleep clinician with complaints of injury to themselves or bed partners. It is normal in REM sleep for the dreamer not to be able to control voluntary muscles. During REM sleep, these muscles are flaccid or atonic.

Otherwise, the dreamer might act out his/her dreams. In RBD this is exactly what happens. The brain mechanism that inhibits muscle activity during dreaming malfunctions and for short periods the dreamer may act out his/her dream. Depending on the content of the dream, this enactment may be dangerous and result in injury to the dreamer or bed partner. RBD research is extremely fast moving especially in light of its recent connection with degenerative brain diseases.[8] Dr Tachibana updates the research as well as diagnostic and treatment issues in her article in this volume.

Despite the rapid advances in research on parasomnias, the lay public, and many doctors, continue to approach sleepwalking and other parasomnias with information that was generally accepted in the 1950s, if not earlier. Sleepwalking remains a mysterious behavior for most individuals. The articles in this volume of *Sleep Medicine Clinics* should serve to bring the reader up to date with the latest data and theories.

As a way of "jump starting" this process, updates concerning a few common misconceptions about parasomnias follow.

1. Sleepwalkers are acting out their dreams.

Prior to the first sleep laboratory studies of sleepwalking in 1965, it was commonly believed that sleepwalkers were acting out their dreams. Starting in 1953, experimental research first described REM. This state was found to be highly correlated with what was commonly called dreaming. The assumption then was that sleepwalking must occur during REM sleep. However, the first sleep studies conducted with sleepwalkers found that sleepwalking did not occur out of REM sleep, but rather followed a partial arousal from deep sleep.

Instead, in 1985, a different sleep disorder in which dreams are enacted was described. RBD is a brain disease in which the brain mechanism that causes muscle tone to be absent during dreaming does not function properly. As a result, voluntary muscle tone is present during dreaming, allowing the dreaming individual to literally act out their dreams. As opposed to sleepwalking that occurs most frequently in children and adolescents, RBD occurs most frequently in older males, many of whom are eventually diagnosed with severe degenerative brain disorders.

2. Sleepwalkers are enacting dreams related to prior psychological traumas.

Sleepwalkers as a group have little or no psychopathology.[9] However, in groups of patients characterized primarily by psychiatric disorders, such as depression, bipolar disease, and anxiety, sleepwalking is reported to be more common than in groups of patients without psychiatric disorders. This increase in sleepwalking behaviors may be related to effects of medications or may indeed not be sleepwalking at all, but the result of central nervous system (CNS) depression during wakefulness.

Sleepwalking appears to be more highly correlated with recent sleep deprivation and situational stress. There is no evidence that chronic stress or depression is correlated with the occurrence of sleepwalking.

Sleepwalking is thought to occur in individuals who have a genetic predisposition for sleepwalking (family history, etc), priming factors, such as sleep deprivation and situational stress, and provoking triggers, such as noise or touch. A "perfect storm" of all three factors is hypothesized to be needed to produce an episode of sleepwalking. Sleepwalking is not a psychological disorder.

3. Sleepwalking is a kind of seizure.

The brain waves (EEG) of sleepwalkers are generally completely normal. Sophisticated brain scans find no tumors, lesions, or other types of brain injury. However, there is evidence that different areas of the brain during sleepwalking function in a dissociated manner. Certain areas that should not be active are active and other areas that should be deactivated or blocked from activating pulses are not. However, seizures and sleepwalking may occur together.

4. Alcohol can trigger sleepwalking.

Severely intoxicated behavior has sometimes been confused with sleepwalking behavior. This was especially so before the modern age of sleep medicine and much was known about the causes of sleepwalking.

Alcohol was initially hypothesized to be related to sleepwalking, because it was said to cause an increase in deep sleep. As noted above, sleep deprivation and increased quantities of deep sleep are a common finding in sleepwalking. However, a recent review of the scientific literature found that in alcohol-naïve or moderate drinkers, alcohol only rarely causes an increase in deep sleep (6 of 19 studies).[10] Additionally, the increase in deep sleep in fact was less than typically noted following sleep deprivation. Further, in individuals who are alcohol abusers or binge drinkers—by far the most common group in whom sleepwalking is said to occur—there is no reported increase in deep sleep.

A search for experimental studies in which alcohol was given to known sleepwalkers in order to determine if it triggered or increased the number of episodes found not a single study.

Thus, the hypothesis of alcohol-induced sleepwalking has no valid evidence-based scientific support and should be considered "junk science." In cases of severe alcohol intoxication, no other explanation for behaviors is required. In most jurisdictions voluntary intoxication is not a complete defense for criminal behavior and in many it provides no justification whatsoever. A suggestion—or legal defense in which alcohol intoxication is reported to cause sleepwalking—often appears to be a way of trying to sidestep the fact that the alcohol intoxication was voluntary and sometime reckless.

"Claims of alcohol-induced parasomnias presented solely to circumvent the laws of voluntary intoxication should be understood for what they are and rejected."[10]

5. Drugs can cause sleepwalking and variants of sleepwalking such as sleep eating and sleep driving.

There are numerous reports of drugs that suppress or depress CNS function, apparently causing sleepwalking and related behaviors in sleep.[11] The use of the term "cause" may not be appropriate as the manner in which drugs and sleepwalking are related has not been established. It is hypothesized that these CNS depressants artificially create a brain state resistant to full arousal. It thus may resemble the brain state following sleep deprivation. It is not known whether individuals susceptible to drug-induced sleepwalking must have a genetic predisposition or not.

Sleeping medications such as zolpidem and zopiclone have been implicated in bizarre, complex behaviors in sleep such as sleep eating and sleep driving.[12] However, they are often combined with painkillers, other sedative hypnotics, and alcohol. Relatively few reports of drug-related complex behaviors in sleep occur following ingestion of a sleeping pill alone. A detailed review of sleep eating can be found in the article by Dr Howell. The relationship of sleep driving to sedative/hypnotic medication may instead be a function of misuse or abuse of sleeping pills. Additionally, it is not clear if sleep driving is a true variant of sleepwalking. In the article by Pressman, the relationship of sleepwalking and medication to sleep driving is reviewed and a new theory is offered.

6. Sleepwalkers generally have amnesia for the episodes, but may retain "islands of memory."

Sleepwalkers generally experience severe anterograde amnesia—meaning they have no memories from the start of the episode until it is finished.

Sleepwalkers don't forget what they did; rather, because of their unusual brain state, they never store the memories. Thus, they will never be able to recall what happened.

Occasionally, if questioned immediately after the episode, sleepwalkers may describe a simple dream-like story. Patients with sleep terrors often begin their episodes with a frightening, but static image, such as "the house was on fire" or "someone was in my room." However, the images typically lack a story or hallucinatory images of dreaming.

The phrase "islands of memory" has been used to describe the residual memory of sleepwalking, has no particular definition, and is not based on experimental research. Attempts to directly test the memory of sleepwalkers during and immediately after episodes have been unsuccessful.[13]

7. Sleepwalkers reenact behaviors or intents from prior wakefulness.

Although this has been suggested by some as a source of sleepwalking behavior, there has been no experimental verification and it appears inconsistent with the general absence of higher cognitive processes including memory during episodes.[14]

8. Waking a sleepwalker in the middle of an episode can cause injury to the sleepwalker.

Sleepwalkers are very hard to awaken. Waking a sleepwalker will cause no harm; however, sleepwalkers may react defensively and violently when they are blocked or touched.[15] The family member or friend who attempts to awaken a sleepwalker during an episode runs the risk of being hit or pushed.

9. Sleepwalkers are violent and seek out victims for revenge.

There is no scientific evidence that sleepwalkers knowingly or voluntarily act violently.[15] There is no evidence that sleepwalkers seek out and attack specific individuals who have caused them harm or damage. Instead, sleepwalkers appear to react instinctively with defensive violence against individuals who are in close proximity to them or who may be perceived as approaching or provoking them. The victim goes to the sleepwalker; the sleepwalker does not seek out the victim.

10. Sleepwalkers have their eyes closed.

Sleepwalkers walk with eyes open. They may navigate more or less successfully in areas that are well known to them; however, their navigation

is not perfect. They may trip over objects in their path or even fall down stairs.

11. Sleepwalking episodes may wax and wane.

Once a sleepwalking episode begins, it continues until it is complete. Sleepwalking only occurs from deep sleep; it cannot occur or recur from wakefulness or light sleep. When a sleepwalking episode ends, it is followed by a brief period of confusion. The confusion is followed by a return to sleep or to full wakefulness.

12. Sleepwalking episodes can last hours.

The overwhelming majority of sleepwalking episodes last only seconds or minutes. However, there have been episodes reported to last an hour or more.[14]

This volume of Sleep Medicine Clinics is devoted to parasomnias, a fascinating and misunderstood sleep disorder that occurs much more frequently than is generally understood. The articles included should allow the reader insight into the different types of parasomnias, state-of-the-art diagnosis, and treatment as well as forensic aspects both past and present.

Mark R. Pressman, PhD, D.ABSM
Sleep Medicine Services
The Lankenau Medical Center and
Lankenau Institute for Medical Research
100 Lancaster Avenue
Wynnewood, PA 19096, USA

E-mail address:
pressmanm@mlhs.org

REFERENCES

1. American Academy of Sleep Medicine. ICSD-2, International classification of sleep disorders. Diagnostic and Coding Manual. 2nd edition. Westchester (IL): American Academy of Sleep Medicine; 2005.

2. Hublin C, Kaprio J. Genetic aspects and genetic epidemiology of parasomnias. Sleep Med Rev 2003;7:413–21.

3. Aserinsky E, Kleitman N. Regularly occurring periods of eye motility, and concomittant phenomena, during sleep. Science 1953;118:273–4.

4. Kales A, Jacobson A, Paulson MJ, et al. Somnambulism: Psychophysiological correlates. I. All-night EEG studies. Arch Gen Psychiatry 1966;14:586–94.

5. Jacobson A, Kales A, Lehmann D, et al. Somnambulism: All-night electroencephalographic studies. Science 1965;975–7.

6. Broughton RJ. Sleep disorders: disorders of arousal? Enuresis, somnambulism, and nightmares

occur in confusional states of arousal, not in "dreaming sleep." Science 1968;159:1070–8.

7. Schenck CH, Bundlie SR, Ettinger MG, et al. Chronic behavioral disorders of human REM sleep: a new category of parasomnia. Sleep 1986;9:293–308.

8. Boeve BF, Silber MH, Saper CB, et al. Pathophysiology of REM sleep behaviour disorder and relevance to neurodegenerative disease. Brain 2007; 130:2770–88.

9. Pressman MR. Factors that predispose, prime and precipitate NREM parasomnias in adults: clinical and forensic implications. Sleep Med Rev 2007;11:5–30.

10. Pressman MR, Mahowald MW, Schenck CS, et al. Alcohol induced sleepwalking or confusional arousals as a defense to criminal behavior: review of scientific evidence, methods and forensic considerations. J Sleep Res 2007;16:198–212.

11. FDA requests label change for all sleep disorder drug products. FDA New Release. Available at: http://www.fda.gov/NewsEvents/Newsroom/PressAnnouncements/2007/ucm108868.htm. Accessed March 14, 2007.

12. Pressman MR. Sleep driving and Z-drugs: Sleepwalking variant or misuse of drugs? Sleep Med Rev 2011, in press.

13. Broughton R. Confusional sleep disorders: interrelationship with memory consolidation and retrieval from sleep. In: Mclean PD, editor. A triune concept of the brain and behavior. Toronto: University of Toronto Press; 1969. p. 115–27.

14. Broughton R, Billings R, Cartwright R, et al. Homicidal somnambulism: a case report. Sleep 1994;17:253–64.

15. Pressman MR. Disorders of arousal from sleep and violent behavior: the role of physical contact and proximity. Sleep 2007;30:1039–47.

State Dissociation: Implications for Sleep and Wakefulness, Consciousness, and Culpability

Mark W. Mahowald, MD[a,b],*,
Michel A. Cramer Bornemann, MD[a,b],
Carlos H. Schenck, MD[c,d]

KEYWORDS

- Consciousness • State dissociation • Sleepwalking
- Sleep terrors • Sleep forensics • Forensic sleep medicine

From a scientific point of view, we can make no distinction between the man who eats little and sees heaven and the man who drinks much and sees snakes.

—Bertrand Russell[1]

This issue of *Sleep Medicine Clinics* explores the fascinating phenomenon of complex behaviors arising from the sleep period, occasionally with dramatic and unfortunate forensic implications. The concept of state dissociation provides a framework for understanding these behaviors and has important implications for consciousness in general. Acknowledgment of the fact that wakefulness/sleep and consciousness/unconsciousness are not mutually exclusive states but rather are characterized by fluid and often fluctuating boundaries will help to explain many curious clinical phenomena and will effect a change in the legal concepts of intent, responsibility, and culpability.

There is now overwhelming evidence that the primary states of being (wakefulness [W], non–rapid eye movement [NREM] sleep, and rapid eye movement [REM] sleep) are not mutually exclusive but may become admixed or may oscillate rapidly resulting in a wide variety of clinical phenomena.[2] Clearly, sleep is a local, and not a global, whole-brain phenomenon.[3–5]

It is likely that, initially, there was only one state of being: (presumably) W. Somewhere and sometime early along the evolutionary trail a second appeared: sleep. Beginning with monotremes, sleep specialized into 2 forms: NREM and REM sleep. Each of these 3 states of being is extremely complex and is composed of numerous physiologic variables, which typically occur in concert, resulting in fully declared states: W, NREM sleep, or REM sleep. The discovery of the bimodal nature of sleep in 1953 launched intense interest in basic science research exploring the nature and pursuing the function of sleep, leading to a dramatic increase in our knowledge of state and state control from neuroanatomic; neurochemical; neurohumoral; neuropharmacologic; neurophysiologic; and, more

This is not an industry-sponsored activity. The authors have no conflict of interest to declare.

[a] Department of Neurology, Minnesota Regional Sleep Disorders Center, Hennepin County Medical Center, 701 Park Avenue, Minneapolis, MN 55415, USA
[b] Department of Neurology, University of Minnesota Medical School, Minneapolis, MN, USA
[c] Department of Psychiatry, Minnesota Regional Sleep Disorders Center, Hennepin County Medical Center, 701 Park Avenue, Minneapolis, MN 55415, USA
[d] Department of Psychiatry, University of Minnesota Medical School, Minneapolis, MN, USA
* Corresponding author. Department of Neurology, Minnesota Regional Sleep Disorders Center, Hennepin County Medical Center, 701 Park Avenue, Minneapolis, MN 55415.
E-mail address: mahow002@umn.edu

recently, molecular genetic aspects. Many of the lessons learned in the process of basic science exploration of state and state control can be readily extrapolated to the human condition, permitting the explanation of bizarre clinical phenomena and leading to effective therapies and a better understanding of conscious awareness.

NORMAL STATE DETERMINATION

The states of W, REM sleep, and NREM sleep are very complex phenomena. State determination may be made using various criteria: behavioral (eyes open/closed, body position, movements, reactivity to the environment); electrographic (electroencephalogram [EEG], electrooculogram, electromyogram [EMG]); or neuronal state (brain neuronal activity). The state-determining properties of each usually cycle in a predictable and uniform manner, resulting in the behavioral appearance of a single prevailing state. However, even in normal individuals, the electrographic and neuronal activity transition among states is gradual and variable, with the simultaneous occurrence or rapid oscillation of multiple state-determining markers (**Fig. 1**).

Furthermore, within each state, there is ongoing variability and fluctuation of central nervous system (CNS) activity.[6,7] The concept of state admixture is hardly new; in his 1963 chapter, "The Onset of Sleep," Nathanial Kleitman described the transition from W to sleep as "a succession of intermediate states, part wakefulness and part sleep in varying proportions - what is designated in Italian as *dormiveglia*, or sleep-waking."[8]

Therefore, the brain undergoes panoramic reorganization as it traverses the 3 states of being. Factors involved in state generation are complex and include a wide variety of neurotransmitters; neuromodulators; neurohormones; and a vast array of sleep factors that act on the multiple neural networks, likely mediated by gene transcription factors.[9,10] There is now good evidence to support the fact that sleep is not necessarily a global, whole-brain phenomenon but a fundamental property of numerous neuronal groups.[4,5,11–13] Therefore, state determination is the result of a dynamic interaction among many variables, including circadian, neural network, neurotransmitter, and myriad sleep-promoting substances and effectors.

The ontogeny of state appearance supports the concept of state dissociation. During embryogenesis, there are no clearly demonstrated states but there is simultaneous admixture of all states, with gradual coalescence resulting in the 3 recognizable states of W/REM/NREM.[14–18] This ontogeny of state development is supported by phylogenetic studies.[19,20] The mechanisms of complex synchronization/recruitment of the state-specific variables are unknown. Basic science neurophysiologists have long known that state dissociation in animals occurs frequently and under many circumstances.[21] The inability of animals to report or indicate mentation and consciousness (ie, waking hallucinations, mental imagery with disorders of arousal, dream-mentation associated motor behavior in REM sleep behavior disorder) has been a significant limitation of the evaluation of animal state dissociation and its application to the human clinical experience.

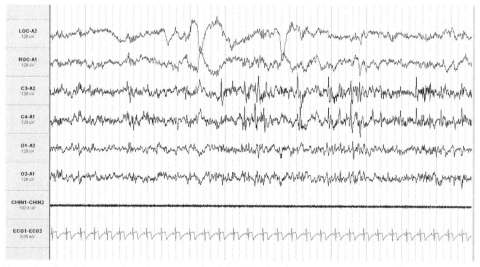

Fig. 1. Example of ambiguous sleep in a normal adult. The simultaneous appearance of rapid eye movements characteristic of REM sleep with sleep spindles/vertex activity characteristic of NREM sleep make state determination difficult. A1, 2: left/right mastoid; C3, 4: left/right central EEG; CHIN, submental EMG; ECG, electrocardiogram; LOC, left outer canthus; O1, 2: left/right occipital EEG; ROC, right outer canthus.

Many endogenous and exogenous factors can affect state cycling/synchronization. These factors include the following[22–24]:

1. Age
2. Sleep deprivation
3. Shift work/rapid travel across time zones
4. Endogenous humoral factors (hormonal)
5. Drugs/medication
6. Affective disorders
7. Environmental stress.

With the multiplicity of state markers and the relatively rapid normal cycling of states requiring recurring recruitment of these numerous physiologic markers, there are innumerable theoretically possible state combinations. Indeed, given the genetic variability of CNS development and its plasticity,[25,26] the relentless cycling, and the ever-present multiplicity of endogenous and environmental influences on both CNS plasticity and cycling, it is actually quite surprising that state-component timing errors do not occur more frequently. Truly, the drive for complete state determination must be very robust.

STATE DISSOCIATION IN ANIMALS

Although the recurrent recruitment of state-determining parameters is amazingly consistent, multiple experimental examples of state component dissociation exist.[27] These experimental dissociations include (1) lesion/stimulation studies, (2) pharmacologic studies, and (3) sleep deprivation studies (for review, see[2]).

In addition to these experimental dissociations, there is evidence in the animal kingdom of the natural occurrence of clinically wakeful behavior during physiologic sleep. Two examples that dispel the concept of all-or-none state declaration are (1) the concurrence of swimming or flight during sleep in birds[28] and (2) the phenomenon of unihemispheric sleep in some aquatic mammals (bottle-nosed dolphin, common porpoise, and northern fur seal) guaranteeing continued respiration while sleeping.[29] Another naturally occurring dissociated state is seen during the arousal from torpor in hibernating ground squirrels, when there is an "uncoupling between thalamic, EMG, and cortical REM correlates."[30]

CLINICAL STATE DISSOCIATION IN HUMANS

Over the centuries, the presentations of and attitudes toward dissociated or automatic behaviors in humans have changed dramatically, ranging from demon possession, witchcraft, shamanism, hysteria, alien abductions, various psychiatric conditions, and frank malingering to the current notion of psychobiologic phenomena. Both experimentally induced and naturally occurring state dissociations in animals serve to predict spontaneously occurring experiments of nature and drug-induced state dissociation in humans, which undoubtedly exist on a very broad spectrum of expression. Such state dissociations are the consequence of timing or switching errors in the normal process of the dynamic reorganization of the CNS as it moves from one state of being to another. Elements of one state persist, or are recruited, erroneously into another state, often with fascinating and dramatic consequences. State dissociations can be thought about in terms of the parent state of W, REM sleep, or NREM sleep.

Dissociation Arising from Wakefulness: Sleepiness

Feelings of sleepiness during W actually represent an admixture or rapid oscillation of W and sleep, a notion exemplified by Dinges' concept that "sleepiness = wake-state instability."[31] Sleepiness is simply the manifestation of an incompletely awake brain.[5,31,32]

Dissociation Arising from Wakefulness: Narcolepsy

Narcolepsy is the prototypic dissociated state arising from the background of W and may best be thought of as a disorder of "state boundary control."[33] The symptom of cataplexy (sudden loss of muscle tone, usually triggered by an emotionally laden event) simply represents the isolated boundary crossing of REM sleep atonia into W. Similarly, the symptom of sleep paralysis is the persistence of REM atonia into W. The hypnagogic (occurring at sleep onset) and hypnopompic (occurring on awakening) hallucinations represent dream mentation occurring during W. Patients with narcolepsy may experience waking dreams (particularly during drowsiness) and be misdiagnosed and even treated as having schizophrenia.[34,35] Importantly, underscoring the tendency to experience switching errors, sleep paralysis and hypnagogic hallucinations occur frequently in the non-narcoleptic population, particularly in the setting of sleep deprivation.[36,37]

Dissociation Arising from NREM Sleep: Disorders of Arousal (Confusional Arousals, Sleepwalking, Sleep Terrors)

Disorders of arousal are the most impressive and most frequent of the NREM sleep-state dissociation/admixture phenomena and are discussed in great detail in article by Banerjee elsewhere in this issue. Disorders of arousal simply represent the simultaneous occurrence of W and NREM sleep. Factors involved in disorders of arousal include sleep inertia and central pattern (locomotor) centers.[2,38] Sleep-related eating disorder and sex-somnia likely represent variations on this theme.[39,40]

Dissociation Arising from REM Sleep: REM Sleep Behavior Disorder

REM sleep behavior disorder (RBD) (discussed in detail in article by Tachibana elsewhere in this issue) is the premier example of a dissociated state arising from the background of REM sleep. The dream-enacting behaviors are allowed to occur because REM sleep is dissociated; all elements of REM sleep are present except atonia (alternatively, one element of W, namely muscle tone, intrudes or persists in REM sleep).[41,42]

Other examples of state dissociation

In addition to simple sleepiness, narcolepsy, disorders of arousal, and RBD, the following phenomena are readily explained by state dissociation[43]:

1. Agrypnia excitata
2. Alien abductions
3. Anesthetic states (conscious sedation)
4. Epic dreaming
5. Hypnagogic/hypnopompic hallucinations
6. Hallucinations (wakeful dreaming)
   a. Charles Bonnet syndrome
   b. Brainstem lesions and musical hallucinations
   c. Phantom limb phenomenon
   d. Peduncular hallucinosis
   e. Neurodegenerative disorders
7. Lucid dreaming
8. Near-death experiences
9. Out-of-body experiences
10. Paradoxic insomnia (formerly sleep state misperception insomnia)
11. Parasomnia overlap syndrome
12. Psychogenic dissociative states
13. Repressed memories of sexual child abuse
14. Sleep inertia
15. Sleep paralysis
16. Status dissociatus.

The increasing numbers of psychiatrists and neurologists practicing sleep medicine will enhance this list as additional previously enigmatic clinical phenomena become explained by differing manifestations of state dissociation.

WHAT CAN SLEEP TEACH US ABOUT CONSCIOUSNESS, AWARENESS, RESPONSIBILITY, AND CULPABILITY?

W and sleep are not global phenomena, but they depend on integration and recruitment of various parts of the nervous system. There is good evidence that the fading of consciousness during certain stages of sleep may be related to a breakdown in cortical effective connectivity. The loss of integration during sleep supports the notion that integration plays a major role in consciousness.

Therefore, W and sleep are analogous to consciousness, which, likewise, depends on the integration and recruitment of various parts of the nervous system.[44]

Anesthesia is making major contributions to the understanding of consciousness. The specific neurophysiologic mechanisms of action of the various anesthetic agents are not known. What is known is that no one mechanism is sufficient to explain how or why the various anesthetic agents produce unconsciousness. It is likely that the mechanisms are varied but result in a final common pathway: disruption of the functional interaction within thalamocortical neural networks.[45]

Numerous names have been applied to this phenomenon including the following:

> State dissociation
> Disjunctive state
> Uncoupling
> Connectivity (functional connectivity)
> Binding (cognitive unbinding)
> Coherence (temporal decoherence)
> Synaptic desynchrony
> Increased connectivity.

As with sleep and W, consciousness is not an all-or-none property, but it increases in proportion to a system's ability to integrate information. Cognitive binding is the proposed mechanism mediating the unity of our experiences. This integration may be dependent on gamma coherence: a widely distributed 30 to 50 Hz rhythm postulated to underlie binding of independent neural assemblies and, thus, integrate processing across distributed neuronal networks to achieve a unified conscious experience. When this rhythm activates both the specific and nonspecific (intralaminar) thalamus simultaneously, different cortical areas are temporally joined and, thus, bound into a single cognitive experience. Binding is the problem of getting together in a single percept such properties as motion, color, outline, and location, which are thought to be detected in different regions of the cortex. Therefore, conscious perception is related to coordinated dynamical states of the cortical network rather than to the activation of specific brain regions.[46–49] During sleep, binding is impaired.[49] Consciousness depends not so much on firing rates, synchronization at specific frequency bands, or sensory input per se but on the brain's ability to integrate information, which is contingent on the effective connectivity among functionally specialized regions of the thalamocortical system.[50]

There is good evidence that unbinding may explain the unconsciousness of sleep.[44,49] The relationship between sleep and anesthesia is further supported by the facts that (1) sleep deprivation reduces the amount of anesthetic agent needed to produce anesthesia and (2) anesthesia lessens the consequences of prior sleep deprivation (anesthesia may count as slow-wave sleep).[51,52] There is an increased requirement for anesthesia in *Drosophila*, with a gene mutation resulting in an extreme reduction in daily sleep requirement.[53]

Cognitive unbinding in other conditions may have relevance to conscious awareness, responsibility, and culpability. Examples include the following:

Thalamocortical dysrhythmia[54]
Schizophrenia[55,56]
Autism[57]
Depression[54]
Drugs (recreational and prescription), drug craving[58,59]
Focal brain lesions[60]
Neurodegenerative disorders.[61]

OTHER EXAMPLES OF DISSOCIATION OF BEHAVIOR AND CONSCIOUSNESS

Such dissociations between behavior and consciousness may be related to inactivation of attentional or memory systems in other conditions.[11]

Alcohol-induced Blackouts

Many forensic cases of sleepwalking defense involve a history of alcohol ingestion. Importantly, alcohol-induced blackouts do not involve loss of consciousness but reflect an isolated disruption of memory for events during a drinking episode. There are 2 types: (1) en bloc or the complete inability to recall events during a circumscribed time period and (2) fragmentary, which is when memory loss is incomplete. Contrary to popular opinion, alcohol-induced blackouts may be seen in individuals who are not problem drinkers and may even occur at the time of one's first drinking experience. The primary determinant of the occurrence of a blackout is not the absolute blood alcohol level (BAL) but the rate of increase of the BAL; blackouts may occur with relatively unimpressive BALs. The explanation for the amnesia

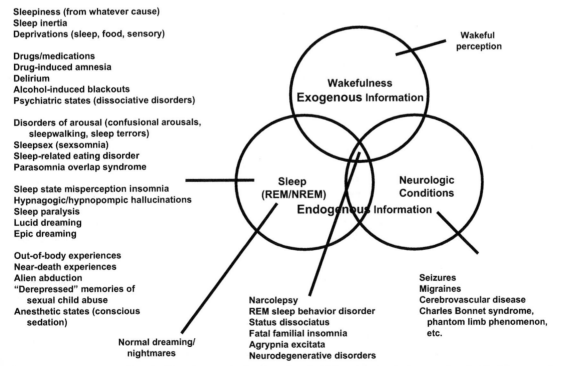

Fig. 2. The spectrum of state dissociations indicating the fluid boundaries between sleep/wakefulness and consciousness/unconsciousness. (*Adapted from* Mahowald MW, Woods SR, Schenck CH. Sleeping dreams, waking hallucinations, and the central nervous system. Dreaming 1998;8:89–102; with permission.)

is a failure of the transfer of short-term memory into long-term storage. The ability to keep information in immediate and short-term memory permits the individual to continue to maintain meaningful conversation. The preferential effect of alcohol on memory before motor impairment explains the high frequency of very complex and elaborate behaviors (driving an automobile, fighting, or sexual experiences) occurring during blackouts without recall.[62] By history, these behaviors may be indistinguishable from those seen in disorders of arousal. In an analogous situation, there is evidence that drug-induced amnesia may be dissociated from drug-induced sedation.[63]

Seizure Activity

The complex behaviors occurring during complex partial seizures and during postictal wanderings (poriomania) likely also represent a disconnection between motor and memory systems.[64–67]

FORENSIC IMPLICATIONS AND OPPORTUNITIES

Aberrant behaviors seen in a wide variety of conditions are likely explained in part by various forms of state dissociation and cognitive unbinding with important forensic implications regarding alertness, awareness, consciousness, intent, culpability, and responsibility (**Fig. 2**). Clearly, W/sleep and consciousness/unconsciousness are graded and not all-or-none, either-or phenomena.[68] Closer collaboration between neuroscientists and the legal community should lead to a better understanding of how best to handle behaviors occurring during dissociated states.

REFERENCES

1. Russell B. Religion and science. New York: Oxford University Press; 1961.
2. Mahowald MW, Schenck CH. Evolving concepts of human state dissociation. Arch Ital Biol 2001;139: 269–300.
3. Rector DM, Schei JL, Van Dongen HP, et al. Physiological markers of local sleep. Eur J Neurosci 2009; 29:1771–8.
4. Nir Y, Staba Richard J, Andrillon T, et al. Regional slow waves and spindles in human sleep. Neuron 2011;70:153–69.
5. Vyazovskiy VV, Olcese U, Hanlon EC, et al. Local sleep in awake rats. Nature 2011;472:443–7.
6. Hobson JA, Scheibel AB. The brainstem core: sensorimotor integration and behavioral state control. Neurosci Res Program Bull 1980;18:1–173.
7. Terzano MG, Parrino L, Spaggiari MC. The cyclic alternating pattern sequences in the dynamic organization of sleep. Electroencephalogr Clin Neurophysiol 1988;69:437–47.
8. Kleitman N. Sleep and wakefulness. Chicago: University of Chicago Press; 1963.
9. Cirelli C, Tononi G. Changes in anti-phosphoserine and anti-phosphothreonine antibody binding during the sleep-waking cycle and after lesion of the locus coeruleus. Sleep Res Online 1998;1:11–8.
10. Tononi G, Cirelli C, Pompeiano M. Changes in gene expression during the sleep-wake cycle: a new view of activating systems. Arch Ital Biol 1995;134:21–37.
11. Hobson JA, Schmajuk NA. Brain state and plasticity: an integration of the reciprocal interaction model of sleep cycle oscillation with attentional models of hippocampal function. Arch Ital Biol 1988;126:209–24.
12. Krueger JM, Obal F Jr, Kapas L, et al. Brain organization and sleep function. Behav Brain Res 1995;69: 177–85.
13. Magnin M, Rey M, Bastuji H, et al. Thalamic deactivation at sleep onset precedes that of the cerebral cortex in humans. Proc Natl Acad Sci U S A 2010; 107:3829–33.
14. Corner MA. Sleep and the beginnings of behavior in the animal kingdom - studies in ultradian motility cycles in early life. Prog Neurobiol 1977;8:279–95.
15. Corner MA. Maturation of sleep mechanism in the central nervous system. Exp Brain Res 1984; 54(Suppl 8):50–66.
16. Corner MA. Ontogeny of brain sleep mechanisms. In: McGinty DJ, Drucker-Colin R, Morrison AR, et al, editors. Brain mechanisms of sleep. New York: Raven Press; 1985. p. 175–97.
17. Corner MA, Bour HL. Postnatal development of spontaneous neuronal discharges in the pontine reticular formation of free-moving rats during sleep and wakefulness. Exp Brain Res 1984;54:66–72.
18. Corner MA. Brainstem control of behavior: ontogenetic aspects. In: Klemm R, Vertes RP, editors. Brainstem mechanisms of behavior. New York: John Wiley & Sons; 1990. p. 239–66.
19. Siegel JM. The evolution of REM sleep. In: Lydic R, Baghdoyan HA, editors. Handbook of behavioral state control cellular and molecular mechanisms. Boca Raton (FL): CRC Press; 1999. p. 87–100.
20. Siegel JM. Phylogeny and the function of REM sleep. Behav Brain Res 1995;69:29–34.
21. Steriade M, Ropert N, Kitsikis A, et al. Ascending activating neuronal networks in midbrain core and related rostral systems. In: Hobson JA, Brazier MA, editors. The reticular formation revisited. New York: Raven Press; 1980. p. 125–67.
22. Inoue S. Biology of sleep substances. Boca Raton (FL): CRC Press; 1989.
23. Anch AM, Browman CP, Mitler MM, et al. Sleep: a scientific perspective. Englewood Cliffs (NJ): Prentice Hall; 1988.

24. Hefez A, Metz L, Lavie P. Long-term effects of extreme situational stress on sleep and dreaming. Am J Psychiatry 1987;144:344–7.

25. Edelman GM. Neural Darwinism. New York: Basic Books; 1987.

26. Fagiolini M, Jensen CL, Champagne FA. Epigenetic influences on brain development and plasticity. Curr Opin Neurobiol 2009;19:207–12.

27. McGinty DJ, Drucker-Colin RR. Sleep mechanisms: biology and control of REM sleep. Int Rev Neurobiol 1982;23:391–436.

28. Amlander CJJ, Ball NJ. Avian sleep. In: Kryger MH, Roth T, Dement WC, editors. Principles and practice of sleep medicine. Philadelphia: W. B. Saunders; 1989. p. 30–49.

29. Zeplin H. Mammalian sleep. In: Kryger MH, Roth T, Dement WC, editors. Principles and practice of sleep medicine. Philadelphia: W. B. Saunders; 1989. p. 30–49.

30. Krilowicz BL, Glotzbach SF, Heller HC. Neuronal activity during sleep and completed bouts of hibernation. Am J Physiol 1988;255:R1008–19.

31. Chuch D, Dinges DF. Mechanisms of sleepiness in obstructive sleep apnea. In: Pack AI, editor. Pathogenesis, diagnosis, and treatment of sleep apnea. New York: Marcel Dekker; 2002. p. 265–85.

32. Van Dongen HP, Belenky G, Krueger JM. A local, bottom-up perspective on sleep deprivation and neurobehavioral performance. Curr Top Med Chem, in press.

33. Broughton R, Valley A, Agquirre M, et al. Excessive daytime sleepiness and the pathophysiology of narcolepsy-cataplexy: a laboratory perspective. Sleep 1986;9:205–15.

34. Shapiro B, Spitz H. Problems in the differential diagnosis of narcolepsy versus schizophrenia. Am J Psychiatry 1976;133:1321–3.

35. Douglass AB, Hays P, Pazderka F, et al. A schizophrenic variant of narcolepsy. Sleep Res 1989;18:173.

36. Takeuchi T, Miyasita A, Sasaki Y, et al. Isolated sleep paralysis elicited by sleep interruption. Sleep 1992; 15:217–25.

37. Ohayon MM, Priest RG, Caulet M, et al. Hypnagogic and hypnopompic hallucinations: pathological phenomena? Br J Psychiatry 1996;169:459–67.

38. Marzano C, Ferrara M, Moroni F, et al. Electroencephalographic sleep inertia of the awakening brain. Neuroscience 2011;176:308–17.

39. Schenck CH, Mahowald MW. Review of nocturnal sleep-related eating disorders. Int J Eat Disord 1994;15:343–56.

40. Schenck CH, Arnulf I, Mahowald MW. Sleep and sex: what can go wrong? A review of the literature on sleep related disorders and abnormal sexual behaviors and experiences. Sleep 2007;30:683–702.

41. Schenck CH, Bundlie SR, Ettinger MG, et al. Chronic behavioral disorders of human REM sleep: a new category of parasomnia. Sleep 1986;9:293–308.

42. Mahowald MW, Schenck CH. REM sleep behavior disorder. In: Kryger MH, Dement W, Roth T, editors. Principles and practice of sleep medicine. 2nd edition. Philadelphia: Saunders; 1994. p. 574–88.

43. Mahowald MW. What state dissociation can teach us about consciousness and the function of sleep [editorial]. Sleep Med 2009;10:159–60.

44. Massimini M, Ferrarelli F, Huber R, et al. Breakdown of cortical effective connectivity during sleep. Science 2005;309:2228–32.

45. White NS, Alkire MT. Impaired thalamocortical connectivity in humans during general-anesthetic-induced unconsciousness. Neuroimage 2003;19: 402–11.

46. Mashour GA. Consciousness unbound. Toward a paradigm of general anesthesia. Anesthesiology 2004;100:428–33.

47. Mashour GA, Forman SA, Campagna JA. Mechanisms of general anesthesia: from molecules to mind. Best Pract Res Clin Anaesthesiol 2005;19: 349–64.

48. Meador KJ, Ray PG, Echauz JR, et al. Gamma coherence and conscious perception. Neurology 2002;59:847–54.

49. Tassi P, Muzet A. Defining states of consciousness. Neurosci Biobehav Rev 2001;25:175–91.

50. Tononi G. The information integration theory of consciousness. In: Max Velmans SS, editor. The Blackwell companion to consciousness. 1st edition. Malden (MA); Oxford (UK); Victoria (Australia): Blackwell Publishing Ltd; 2007. p. 287–99.

51. Nelson AB, Faraguna U, Tononi G, et al. Effects of anesthesia on the response to sleep deprivation. Sleep 2010;33:1659–67.

52. Allada R. An emerging link between general anesthesia and sleep. Proc Natl Acad Sci U S A 2008; 105:2257–8.

53. Weber B, Schaper C, Bushey D, et al. Increased volatile anesthetic requirement in short-sleeping drosophila mutants. Anesthesiology 2009;110: 313–6.

54. Llinas RR, Ribary U, Jeanmonod D, et al. Thalamocortical dysrhythmia: a neurological and neuropsychiatric syndrome characterized by magnetoencephalography. Proc Natl Acad Sci U S A 1999;96:15222–7.

55. Vercammen A, Knegtering H, den Boer JA, et al. Auditory hallucinations in schizophrenia are associated with reduced functional connectivity of the temporo-parietal area. Biol Psychiatry 2010;67: 912–8.

56. Pettersson-Yeo W, Allen P, Benetti S, et al. Dysconnectivity in schizophrenia: where are we now? Neurosci Biobehav Rev 2011;35:1110–24.

57. Redcay E, Courchesne E. Deviant functional magnetic resonance imaging patterns of brain activity to speech in 2-3-year-old children with autism spectrum disorder. Biol Psychiatry 2008;64:589–98.

58. Fingelkurts AA, Fingelkurts AA, Kivisarri R, et al. Opioid withdrawal results in increased local and remote functional connectivity at EEG alpha and beta frequency bands. Neurosci Res 2007;58: 40–9.

59. Kelly C, Zuo XN, Gotimer K, et al. Reduced inter-hemispheric resting state functional connectivity in cocaine addiction. Biol Psychiatry 2011;69: 684–92.

60. Bartolomei F, Bosma I, Klein M, et al. How do brain tumors alter functional connectivity? A magnetoencephalographic study. Ann Neurol 2006;59: 128–38.

61. Seeley WW, Crawford RK, Zhou J, et al. Neurodegenerative diseases target large-scale human brain networks. Neuron 2009;62:42–52.

62. Rose ME, Grant JE. Alcohol-induced blackout. Phenomenology, biological basis, and gender differences. J Addict Med 2010;4:61–73.

63. Veselis RA, Reinsel RA, Feshchenko VA. Drug-induced amnesia is a separate phenomenon from sedation. Anesthesiology 2001;95:896–907.

64. Licht EA, Fujikawa DG. Nonconvulsive status epilepticus with frontal features: quantitating severity of subclinical epileptiform discharges provides a marker for treatment efficacy, recurrence and outcome. Epilepsy Res 2002;51:13–21.

65. Chang AK, Shinnar S. Nonconvulsive status epilepticus. Emerg Med Clin North Am 2011;29:65–72.

66. Shorvon S, Trinka E. Nonconvulsive status epilepticus and the postictal state. Epilepsy Behav 2010;19:172–5.

67. De Tiege X, Ligot N, Goldman S, et al. Metabolic evidence for remote inhibition in epilepsies with continuous spike-waves during sleep. Neuroimage 2008;40:802–10.

68. Nir Y, Tononi G. Dreaming and the brain: from phenomenology to neurophysiology. Trends Cogn Sci 2010;14:88–100.

Sleepwalking

Dev Banerjee, MBChB, MD, FRCP[a,b,*],
Angus Nisbet, BMedSci, BM, BS, FRCP[c]

KEYWORDS

- Sleepwalking • Somnambulism
- Slow-wave arousal disorder • Parasomnia

Since his majesty went into the field, I have seen her rise from her bed, throw her nightgown upon her, unlock her closet, take forth paper, fold it, write upon't, read it, afterwards seal it, and again return to bed; yet all this while in a most fast sleep. ....[ ]....You see, her eyes are open. ...[]....Ay, but their sense is shut. ...[]....Look, how she rubs her hands. ....[ ]....I have known her continue in this a quarter of an hour. ....[ ]... Yet here's a spot. ...[ ].... Hark! she speaks. ....[ ]... Out, damned spot! out, I say!—One: two: why, then, 'tis time to do't.—Hell is murky!— Fie, my lord, fie! a soldier, and afeard? What need we fear who knows it, when none can call our power to account?—Yet who would have thought the old man to have had so much blood in him?

—William Shakespeare Macbeth Act 5, Scene 1

Shakespeare attributed Lady Macbeth's sleepwalking episodes to a combination of her overwhelming grief and to "insanity." But the mysteries of sleepwalking have not only interested the minds of great writers but also composers such as Vincenzo Bellini, whose opera *La Somnambula* is named after its heroine, a sleepwalker, and more recently filmmakers such as Walt Disney (*Sleepy-Time Donald*, 1947) and Alfonso Cuaron's *Harry Potter and the Prisoner of Azkaban* (2004) in which Harry Potter uses sleepwalking as an excuse as to why he was out of bed after hours. This article reviews the scientific literature on the subject of sleepwalking, with the aim of better understanding and attempting to unravel the mysteries of this fascinating condition.

NEUROPHYSIOLOGY OF SLEEPWALKING

Sleepwalking and related disorders are not, as is commonly thought, enacted dreams. Sleepwalking does not occur from rapid-eye-movement (REM) sleep but rather occurs following a partial arousal from deep or slow-wave sleep (SWS). Because sleepwalking and related disorders follow a partial arousal, they are often called disorders of arousal. Sleepwalking/confusional arousals and night terrors are disorders of SWS arousal.[1] **Fig. 1** shows a polysomnograph (PSG) of a sudden arousal during SWS presenting as a confusional arousal in the sleep laboratory of author A.N. There has been considerable debate on the functional abnormalities of SWS in those who sleepwalk. An early study confirmed that somnambulistic episodes in sleepwalking occurred in non-REM sleep, predominantly in SWS,[2] but not necessarily confined to the first third of the night. Evaluation of SWS in sleepwalkers have shown that more time is spent in SWS, with more SWS interruptions seen.[3] Although nonspecific, the investigators speculate that such findings on the PSG may assist in the clinical diagnosis.[4]

The authors have nothing to disclose.

[a] Academic Department of Sleep and Ventilation, Birmingham Heartlands Hospital, Heart of England NHS Foundation Trust, Bordesley Green East, B9 5SS Birmingham, UK

[b] Aston Brain Centre, School of Life and Health Sciences, Aston University, B4 7ET Birmingham, UK

[c] East Grinstead Sleep Disorders Centre, Queen Victoria Hospital NHS Foundation Trust, London Road, East Grinstead, West Sussex RH19 1QE, UK

* Corresponding author. Academic Department of Sleep and Ventilation, Birmingham Heartlands Hospital, Heart of England NHS Foundation Trust, Bordesley Green East, Birmingham, UK.

E-mail address: Dev.banerjee@heartofengland.nhs.uk

Sleep Med Clin 6 (2011) 401–416

doi:10.1016/j.jsmc.2011.07.001

A

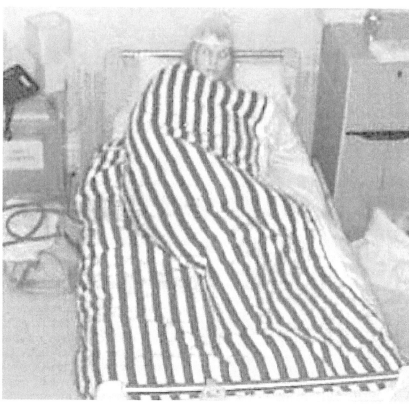

Fig. 1. (*A*) The patient, a 46-year-old married female teaching assistant attending the sleep clinic for a consultation with author A.N., sits up suddenly during slow-wave sleep in the sleep laboratory. She had been sleepwalking from before the age of 10 years and regularly from then on. The exact age of onset was unknown. Over the last year, the frequency of sleepwalking had increased from once per week to almost every night, usually once per night but sometimes up to 3 times per night. There was no family history of sleepwalking. No specific triggers were identified in the patient's history. All episodes begin with her suddenly sitting bolt upright in bed. At this point she recalls marked anxiety, which she describes as "half aware" and with a strong sense of having to do something or be somewhere—she cannot recall what or where. Her eyes are open as witnessed by her husband. There are never vivid dreams or hallucinations. The majority of episodes (>90%) involve ambulation. Automatic activity has been noted, particularly repeatedly opening a particular wardrobe, checking the bathroom, checking on the children, going downstairs to check other rooms, and opening curtains. The onset of most episodes is also accompanied by vocalization during which she characteristically shouts out "oh my God" or similar phrases in a panicky voice. She often wails loudly but rarely screams. If talked to by her partner she answers in a defensive and argumentative fashion and does not seem to take in what she is told. On rare occasions she has hit her partner. No eating or sexual behavior has been observed. The episodes last about 5 minutes but range between 1 and 15 minutes. Episodes are more likely to occur if she is away from home or stressed, but are not influenced by the amount of sleep she gets. She complains of chronically unrefreshing sleep and chronic daytime fatigue, and although she has a regular afternoon nap she scored 7 out of 24 on the ESS. She is not easily awoken, especially in the mornings. She has no insomnia symptoms and there is no history of hypnic jerks, leg movements, or snoring, There is no history of sleep paralysis and no history of hypnagogic or hypnopompic hallucinations, and no lucid dreaming. Her magnetic resonance imaging brain scan was normal. A single night's polysomnography recording revealed two episodes of paroxysmal confusional arousal in which she sat up in bed and vocalized. Both episodes lasted less than a minute. The first occurred in typical stage 2 sleep during which she uttered "oh my God." The second occurred in slow-wave sleep (*B*), lasting longer, and was accompanied by a vocalization in which she said "hang on a minute" followed by something else indecipherable. This episode terminated the first cycle of slow-wave sleep, which was her most sustained period of slow-wave sleep with highest delta power. There were no clear triggers to either episode. She had excessive microarousals throughout all sleep stages (arousal index was 23 events per hour using American Academy of Sleep Medicine rules). Cyclic alternative patterns were frequent throughout non-REM sleep. Apnea-hypopnea index was 2.6 per hour of sleep, periodic leg movement index was less than 2 events per hour of sleep, and the isolated limb movement index was 6.8 per hour of sleep. A diagnosis of non-REM arousal parasomnia was made.

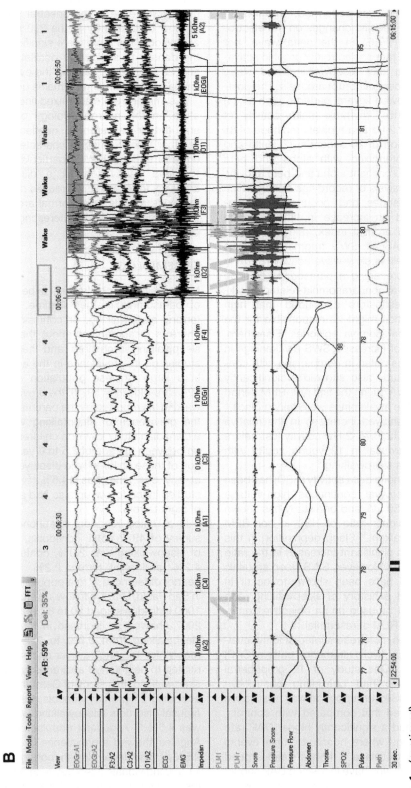

Fig. 1. (*continued*)

In a study of 38 adult sleepwalkers with or without sleep terrors, detailed analysis of 252 arousals from SWS was performed.[5] The investigators found no specific changes on the electroencephalograph (EEG) in the delta wave, nor changes in heart rate or electromyographic activation, concluding that sleepwalking and sleep terrors are disorders of abrupt arousals. The postarousal EEG showed several patterns such as: (1) mixture of diffuse, rhythmic delta activity of a frequency of 2.2 Hz and typical amplitude of 85 μV with a duration of 20 seconds; (2) delta and theta activity intermixed with alpha and beta activity; and (3) prominent alpha and beta activity. Another PSG analysis of recordings during which parasomnia episodes had occurred in sleepwalkers showed an increase in time spent in SWS, increased arousal index, and wake after sleep onset (WASO).[6] SWS fragmentation was prominent as well as slow-wave activity (SWA) in the 2 minutes preceding a parasomnia episode compared with a nonparasomnia-related awakening. The investigators concluded that high SWS fragmentation might be responsible for the occurrence of parasomnia episodes. Elsewhere, the occurrence of increased SWS awakenings in sleepwalkers was noted in comparison with controls, but this study also showed a significantly lower level of SWA during the first non-REM period when most of the awakenings were taking place.[7] Another study showed increases in the relative power of low delta (0.75–2 Hz) activity just before a confusional arousal in 12 young adults with known long-term sleepwalking.[8]

Hypersynchronous delta activity (HSD) has been described as several continuous high-voltage delta waves (≥150 μV), and one study has shown a significantly higher ratio of HSD in non-REM sleep of sleepwalkers.[9] Sleep deprivation in this study resulted in significant increases in the ratio of the time in HSD. However, SWS sleep arousals and HSD sleep have been shown to occur in subjects without a history of sleepwalking, and therefore cannot be used as an objective confirmation of a non-REM parasomnial.[10]

There has been more recent interest in the evaluation of non-REM cyclic alternation pattern (CAP) in sleepwalkers. One study of 12 prepubertal sleepwalkers who had coexisting obstructive sleep apnea (OSA) or upper airway resistance syndrome showed that compared with controls, sleepwalkers had a significantly higher CAP rate during recordings where nonparasomnia events (eg, apneas) took place.[11] It has been argued that sleepwalkers who have increased CAP should be considered as possibly having other sleep-breathing disorders.[12]

A further study looking at SWA before somnambulistic episodes showed that there was no gradual increase in the spectral power for delta or slow delta activity in the 200 seconds before an episode, but there were significant changes in the density of slow-wave oscillations during the final 20 seconds preceding the event.[13] The relevance of these findings remains unclear.

In summary, there are mixed findings in the literature on the neurophysiology of sleepwalking, and further research is needed to determine whether sleepwalking is characterized by a disorder of abnormal SWS, particularly its response to sleep deprivation, or a disorder of SWS arousals, for example, increased number of spontaneous arousals or abnormal arousal response. Further research in this interesting field has been called for.[14]

EPIDEMIOLOGY

Many preschool children will experience one form of parasomnia in their lifetime, such as night terrors, sleepwalking, or confusional arousals.[15] There is disagreement about the prevalence of sleepwalking in children, and there are very few studies on its prevalence in the adult population. In a large Chinese population study of 2- to 12-years-olds (n = 5979), the prevalence of sleepwalking, as reported by the parents, was 0.6% and the prevalence of sleeptalking was 4.9%.[16] In a Canadian study in which children were followed up between the age of 2.5 to 6 years, the proportion of these children who displayed sleepwalking at any one time was 14.5%.[17] Those children studied in the follow-up also had a high incidence of night terrors.

In a United Kingdom telephone questionnaire survey of 4972 adult individuals, the prevalence of sleepwalking was 2.0%, confusional arousals 4.2%, and night terrors 2.2%. There were no gender differences.[18] In a population-based study in São Paulo, Brazil, a follow-up study of more than 1000 individuals aged 20 to 80 years from 1987 to 2007 showed an increase in the prevalence of sleepwalking from 0.8% to 2.8%.[19] The exact reason for this increase is unclear, but may be related to heightened awareness and reporting of sleepwalking. In a study of German schoolchildren attending 27 primary schools, the prevalence of arousal disorders (sleepwalking and night terrors) was 4.6%.[20] A general population survey in Los Angeles showed a prevalence of sleepwalking of 2.5%,[21] and in a Finnish cohort of more than 11,000 individuals aged between 33 and 60 years, the prevalence of frequent sleepwalking in childhood was higher in women than in men (2.8% vs

2.0%), but as adults, men were more likely to sleepwalk than women (3.9% vs 3.1%).[22] Those who reported walking in their sleep often or sometimes in childhood did so as adults in 24.6% of men and in 18.3% of women. Of the adult male sleepwalkers, 88.9% had a positive history of sleepwalking in their childhood, and in women this was 84.5%. Those who reported never to have walked in their sleep in childhood did so rarely in adulthood (0.6%), and this was similar for both genders.

Canadian data have also shown that the prevalence of sleepwalking declines as children get older, including other parasomnias, for example, body rocking and night terrors.[23] There was no gender difference seen for sleepwalking in this study. Overall these studies suggest that sleepwalking is not rare, but these epidemiologic studies were performed on populations of interest, and in studies of children were based on parental recall. Therefore, such data cannot be accurately extrapolated to the whole population and thus the true prevalence remains unknown. Few studies have also assessed the frequency of sleepwalking during the night and how this may vary with different geographic populations and ethnicity.

FAMILY TRAITS AND GENETICS

Anecdotally, sleep experts report positive family histories of sleepwalking or sleep terrors in first-degree relatives of sleepwalking patients attending their clinics. Recently there has been an increased interest in the genetics of sleepwalking. In one study of 7 families, 50 close family relatives were questioned and 34 of whom were identified as having a history of sleepwalking.[24] In a large Finnish twin cohort of more than 11,000 people including 1045 monozygotic and 1899 dizygotic twin pairs, there was no significant difference in the frequency of sleepwalking between monozygotic and dizygotic twin individuals, either in childhood or in adulthood.[22] A 4-generation family was studied whereby 9 of the affected and 13 of the unaffected family members were interviewed with DNA samples collected for parametric linkage analysis.[25] The investigators concluded that in this family, sleepwalking was inherited as an autosomal dominant disorder with reduced penetrance, and that there was a genetic locus for sleepwalking at chromosome 20q12-q13.12. Certainly these findings are intriguing, and may stimulate further research aimed at confirming that there is indeed a genetic link to explain the familial tendencies. However, it may be some time before the full understanding of the genetic

makeup of sleepwalking is unraveled and its potential uses (eg, screening and diagnostic validity) become routine.[26]

CLINICAL FEATURES

The term parasomnia is commonly used to denote undesirable physical and behavioral phenomena occurring during sleep. However, the clinical features of sleepwalking remain varied, and can range from simple confusional arousals and brief episodes of sleepwalking in young children to night terrors and dramatic episodes of sleep running accompanied by screaming. Other types of automatic behavior, especially instinctual behavior, can be seen in those who sleepwalk, including sleep-related eating (see the article by Howell elsewhere in this issue), violence, and sexual activity (see the article by Buchanan elsewhere in this issue). Many have features of several of these phenomena during their lives, with behavioral patterns evolving from night terrors when a child, to sleepwalking as a teenager, to confusional arousals as an adult, or a mixture of all 3 of these parasomnia-like forms occurring throughout life.[27,28] Sitting bolt upright or running is usually accompanied by panicky vocalizations and, in extreme cases, screaming, and hence is considered to be a combination of a sleep terror and sleepwalking. Most of the actions are simple, crude even. The behaviors that are performed by a sleepwalker are not regarded as in keeping with sophisticated cognitive behaviors such as memory, intent, planning, or social interaction.[29] However, the particular spectrum of behavior seen may depend on which areas of the cortex are aroused and which are still in SWS,[30] and which areas are activated and deactivated, as seen in a reported case of a sleepwalker undergoing single-photon emission computed tomography (SPECT).[31]

In an analysis of 39 (21 males) consecutive patients attending an adult sleep clinic (A. Nisbet, unpublished data, 2011), the majority of patients commenced sleepwalking in childhood and 38% had a history of a first-degree sleepwalking relative (**Table 1**). Running or escaping was the most common behavior described (**Table 2**), followed by other automatic behaviors (other than walking or sitting up). The incidence of sleep violence (36%) and sleep sexual activity (13%) may be overrepresented in this group because of a referral bias, as population-based studies are more reliable in ascertaining the precise incidence. However, these figures may reflect a typical sleep clinic population of sleepwalkers. Automatic activity other than walking, running, or sitting up was found to be very common in this group, as

Table 1
Characteristics of 39 (21 males) consecutive patients with a history of sleepwalking attending an adult sleep clinic

Mean (range) age at first consultation (y)	32.7 (17–59)
Mean (range) age of onset (y)	16.0 (3–40)
Mean (range) number of active parasomnia nights (per mo)	10.4 (0.2–30)
Mean (range) frequency of events during active nights (per night)	1.6 (1–10)
History of childhood (<10 y) non-REM parasomnia	69%
History of a first degree relative with non-REM parasomnia	38%
History of PTSD/abuse/major psychological trauma[a]	15%

Abbreviation: PTSD, posttraumatic stress disorder.
[a] Data missing in 12.

Table 2
Characteristics of nocturnal behavior during sleep in 39 (21 males) consecutive patients with a history of sleepwalking attending an adult sleep clinic

Behavior	Frequency
Running or escaping	51%
Screaming	21%
Physical aggression directed toward another person	36%
Eating	5%
Sexual activity	13%
Dressing	8%
Any automatic behavior (other than walking or sitting up)	46%
REM Parasomnic Phenomena	
Nightmares	10%
Sleep paralysis	8%
Subjective Sleep Parameters	
Features of insomnia including difficulty initiating and maintaining sleep	13%
Unrefreshing sleep[a]	49%
Mean (range) ESS	7.2 (0–19)

Abbreviation: ESS, Epworth Sleepiness Scale.
[a] Data missing in 4.

was escape behavior (46%). Escape behavior was surprisingly common (51%) as was screaming (21%), that is, night terrors (but not necessarily featured during walking arousals). In fact, some degree of apprehension was a common feature of the nocturnal arousals. It is interesting that although the Epworth Sleepiness Scale (ESS) was generally within a normal range for a population without other sleep disorders, these patients commonly reported unrefreshing sleep (49%), especially during periods when the sleepwalking or other associated non-REM arousals were frequent. A recent study of 10 sleepwalking individuals in fact showed objective sleepiness using the Multiple Sleep Latency Test (MSLT) compared with controls, indicating possibly that sleepwalkers are sleepier than those who do not sleepwalk.[32]

In a study of children between the age of 2 and 12 years, those with parasomnias had higher prevalence of bedtime resistance, sleep-onset delay, night waking, and reduced sleep duration compared with a matched sample without reported parasomnia. One-quarter of these sleepwalkers also reported nocturnal enuresis.[33]

There has been debate on whether those who sleepwalk have dreamlike experiences. In a recent retrospective survey study of 43 patients with both sleepwalking and night terrors, 71% did recall imagery that they associated with previous parasomnias. These images were usually unpleasant with the individual being the victim of aggression in 24%, misfortune in 54%, or apprehension in 84% in those who did have recall.[34] However, the retrospective and anecdotal character of these descriptions along with the anterograde amnesia common in non-REM parasomnia suggest these data should not be accepted at face value. The investigators hypothesized that sleepwalking may act out corresponding dreamlike mentation. However, it remains unclear whether any complex cognition such as dreaming could occur simultaneously with generalized SWA and whether such dreamlike experiences arise later during the course of the parasomnia. There has also been a suggestion that trauma-recall associations during sleepwalking may be linked to previous major psychological trauma.[35] The authors' case series would lend some support to this contention, with a history of posttraumatic stress disorder (PTSD), abuse, or major psychological trauma seen in a proportion of the sleepwalking cohort. How these psychological factors influence the parasomnia episode is unclear, but it may be hypothesized that such psychological factors may be related to images or mentation that takes place after the onset of the arousal, and that it is the arousal that is the prime mover. However, it is generally accepted that sleepwalkers as a group do not have significant psychopathology. The family history and childhood onset that have been described in many sleepwalkers is consistent with an arousal tendency that may arise from genetically predisposed individuals.

MODIFYING FACTORS, PRIMERS, AND TRIGGERS

The predisposition (genetically) of sleepwalking has already been discussed here, but the key to assessing a sleepwalking case clinically is the assessment of modifying, priming, and precipitating triggers. A detailed review of this has been published previously, particularly the clinical and forensic implications.[36] Although a predisposition to sleepwalking may be present, such events may only occur when priming and precipitating factors are also present. Some factors may deepen sleep or make full and rapid arousal from sleep more difficult, as well as promote fragmentation of sleep or increase the chances of sleepwalking episodes in those who are genetically predisposed (see the article by Zadra and Pilon in this issue).[36] One study of 10 sleepwalkers who underwent 38 hours of sleep deprivation found a significant increase in the frequency and complexity of sleepwalking episodes during the recovery night compared with baseline.[37] Another study assessed the induction of somnambulistic episodes by sleep deprivation and forced arousals (auditory stimuli). No somnambulistic episodes were induced in nonsleepwalkers. All those who underwent 25 hours of sleep deprivation experienced at least one induced episode of somnambulistic episode during the recovery SWS as compared with normal SWS (30%).[38] The same group also reported that sleep deprivation in a sleep laboratory led to a more successful documentation of somnambulistic episodes in those with known sleepwalking, as a result of the increased homeostatic pressure for sleep.[39] These studies confirm that those predisposed to sleepwalking can have episodes induced in a controlled manner, and the investigators suggest that the development of such protocols (ie, sleep deprivation followed by forced arousals) in the sleep laboratory may help the establishment of a video-PSG confirmation of diagnosis.

Another predisposing factor to consider is alcohol. Alcohol has been included in many previously published lists of potential predisposing or triggering factors for sleepwalking, although no experimental research exists to support this theory. Alcohol-related behaviors are also often confused with sleepwalking by the lay public. However, a recent review of the literature concluded that there is no direct experimental evidence that alcohol predisposes or triggers sleepwalking.[40,41] Further, there is little research to support the theory that alcohol is related to sleepwalking because it causes an increase in SWS. The role of sleep-disordered breathing and restless legs with periodic leg movements as a trigger is discussed later. One study has shown that the frequency of sleepwalking is reduced during pregnancy, more so in the primiparous than in the multiparous group.[42]

SLEEPWALKING AND INJURIOUS BEHAVIOR

Injurious and violent behavior during sleep (VBS) is not rare, and in a European study of nearly 20,000 participants undergoing an epidemiologic questionnaire on this subject, up to 1.6% reported such nocturnal behaviors.[43] Up to 4 in 5 reported vivid dreams and more than 30% sustained injuries, with a family history reported more frequently in those with VBS than in those without. The highest odds for violent behavior were associated with sleepwalking and night terrors (73%). In another study of 100 consecutive adults presenting to a sleep clinic complaining of repeated nocturnal injury, PSG suggested sleepwalking and night terrors in 54 subjects, REM behavior disorder (RBD) in 36, dissociative disorders in 7, seizures in 2, and OSA in 1.[44] Sustained bruising was seen in 95% of the subjects, 30 had lacerations, and 9 had fractures.

Nocturnal wandering during sleepwalking can be associated with self-inflicted injuries.[45] Some of the injuries can be mistaken for an intentional self-injury episode.[46] In addition, some deaths ruled as suicides may instead be related to the consequence of sleep-related complex behavior without premeditation and conscious awareness.[47] In a study of 41 subjects with nocturnal wandering (age group between 12 and 63 years), 29 subjects reported injuries, either to themselves or to others, with arousals from sleep triggered in some by sleep-disordered breathing.[48] Indeed in one of the authors' (A.N.) case series, sleep-related aggression directed toward another person occurred in a large proportion of sleepwalkers (36%).

However, not all violence during sleep can be assigned directly to sleepwalking, and the sleep expert must be aware that violence may be related to dissociative disorders, malingering, and Munchausen syndrome by proxy[49] during periods of full wakefulness occurring during sleep. Violent behavior directed against another individual usually follows direct triggering by or close proximity to another individual.[50] Sleepwalkers generally do not seek out their victims; rather, victims seek or are encountered by the sleepwalker.[50] Certainly this is an area of much legal debate, and there have been cases of acquittal on the basis of sleepwalking constituting the legal defense.[51] Men are more likely to commit serious violent acts, and drug and alcohol abuse is not uncommon.[52] One published case is of a 43-year-old man who would undertake frenzied running, throwing punches and wielding knives.[53] This case report also described the sleepwalker as driving an automobile for a long distance in a presumed somnambulistic state (see the article Pressman elsewhere in this issue). PSG confirmed multiple episodes of complex and violent behaviors arising from SWS. The patient responded well to clonazepam.

It is now recognized that sleep specialists are being asked more often to provide opinions and judgments on legal cases of possible sleepwalking-related violence for which the defense is a legal automatism.[54–57] The assessment of how exactly to approach such a legal case in the sleep laboratory (including the pros and cons of PSG) continues to be debated in sleep medicine.[58] However, it is generally accepted that PSG performed after the fact cannot assist in determining whether a defendant performed a violent or criminal act in the midst of a sleepwalking episode.[36,56]

SLEEPWALKING AND SEXUAL BEHAVIOR

There is a growing awareness of abnormal sexual behavior emerging during sleep and, as such, terms such as "sleepsex" or "sexsomnia" have been coined to describe these activities (see the article by Buchanan elsewhere in this issue).[59] Sleep sex has been used as the basis of a legal defense for rape and sexual misconduct.[60,61] Recently a detailed literature review has been undertaken to classify these behaviors.[62] Sexual behaviors specific to parasomnias include sexual vocalization/talking/shouting, masturbation, fondling another person, sexual intercourse with or without orgasm, and agitated or assaultive sexual behavior.[62] A history of sleepwalking and confusional arousals is often found to be present in those who have exhibited sexsomnia. Men are reported to make up 80% of the case series of parasomnia-related sexsomnia, with an average age of 32 years. Fondling and sexual intercourse were the most common activities, and memory recall was not recorded in any of the cases. Clonazepam was the most common medication used, and proved effective in the majority. It was rare to exhibit sexsomnia without a history of other parasomnias. There are very few cases of reported sleep-related sexual activity during in-laboratory PSG in the literature.

ASSOCIATION OF SLEEPWALKING WITH OTHER SLEEP DISORDERS

Assessment of sleepwalking patients may uncover the concomitant presence of other sleep disorders. A telephone interview study of 4972 individuals in the United Kingdom showed that subjects who sleepwalk (2.0% prevalence) had an increased prevalence of self-reported apneas and choking at night.[18] In a study of 84 prepubertal children with sleepwalking and/or night terrors, 49 had sleep-disordered breathing and 2 had restless legs syndrome with periodic limb movements during sleep.[63] Of the 49 with sleep-disordered breathing, 47 were treated with tonsillectomy, adenoidectomy, and/or turbinate revision. Of these, 43 showed resolution of sleep-disordered breathing and an improvement in SWS arousal frequency as seen on a follow-up PSG. In those for whom sleep-disordered breathing improved, there was also an associated absence of further parasomnia episodes. The 2 cases with restless legs syndrome and periodic leg movements were treated with pramipexole, a dopamine agonist at bedtime, with documented improvement in periodic leg movement frequency from a follow-up PSG, and also an improvement in the frequency of parasomnia episodes. The investigators concluded that sleep-disordered breathing and restless legs syndrome with periodic leg movements may be a trigger of non-REM parasomnias in children.

The importance of looking for coexisting OSA and periodic leg movements in sleepwalking patients cannot be overemphasized.[18,64,65] Treatment of OSA with continuous positive airway pressure has also been shown to resolve sleepwalking,[65] and this was also related to the degree of compliance with therapy. Those who were noncompliant continued to sleepwalk. The link between restless legs syndrome as a coexisting sleep disorder with sleepwalking has been reported elsewhere.[66]

SLEEPWALKING AND EATING

There have been reports that sleep-related eating (SRE) (see the article by Howell elsewhere in this issues) is a common feature of sleepwalkers, and in one study of 19 adults presenting to a sleep clinic with sleep SRE, 84% were sleepwalkers.[67] Another 10% had periodic leg movements during sleep. Onset of SRE was linked with the onset of the sleep disorder. Nearly three-quarters were women, and the average age onset was 24 years. More than half ate nightly and the chief complaints were excessive weight gain, concerns about choking, and the use of gas fires for cooking.

However, it cannot be assumed that all nocturnal eating is related to sleep. In 35 consecutive patients presenting to a sleep center with nocturnal eating who underwent detailed PSG, 45 episodes of nocturnal eating were documented in 26 patients, and eating always occurred after complete awakening from non-REM sleep except for only one who awoke from REM sleep.[68] Significant numbers of periodic limb movements were recorded in 22 patients. Recurrent chewing and swallowing movements occurred in 29 patients. The investigators hypothesize that compulsory food-seeking behavior may have a dopaminergic dysfunction in origin. In another study of 23 consecutive cases with SRE, it was found that 11 (48%) had a history of sleepwalking and that 8 (35%) had a lifetime eating disorder diagnosis.[69] The majority of this cohort was women. More than 90% of the cohort described their sleep state as either "asleep" or "half awake/half asleep." The treatment of SRE is discussed later.

SLEEPWALKING AND PSYCHIATRIC DISORDERS

The role of the mind in sleepwalking has been debated for many years. An early study found an increased level of "hysteria" and anxiety in sleepwalkers.[70] A Hong Kong study, however, highlighted an 8.5% prevalence rate of sleepwalking in a large psychiatric outpatient clinic.[71] The same group also reported a higher usage of zolpidem for insomnia symptoms in this sleepwalking group.[72] However, little or no psychopathology has been reported in patients with a primary complaint of sleepwalking. Childhood sleep problems have been documented to be associated with perinatal risk factors, parental psychopathology, and children's behavioral issues.[73] However, sleep disturbances have been reported to be common in children with attention deficit/hyperactivity disorder (ADHD), with one study of 55 children (47 were boys) with average age 8.9 years finding that sleepwalking was noted by parents in nearly half of the cohort (48%), night terrors in 38%, and confusional arousals in 28%.[74] A separate study has found an increase in neurosis in sleepwalkers.[75]

SLEEPWALKING AND OTHER MEDICAL CONDITIONS

The prevalence of sleepwalking in other medical conditions has not been reported widely. Sleep-walking has been shown to have a prevalence of 2.1% in a cohort of 883 dialysis patients.[76] Although RBDs have been commonly described in those with Parkinson Disease (PD), sleepwalking in PD is not common; occurring as de novo adult-onset sleepwalking in 4% in two reported studies.[77,78] These patients also reported a higher prevalence of hallucinations and nightmares, and associated RBD. There has been a reported higher prevalence of sleepwalking in patients with vitiligo. Although the investigators speculate a serotoninergic neural mechanism for this link, there have been no other similar reports of such an association.[79] There have been reports of sleepwalking in patients with dementia, with a prevalence of up to 0.5%.[80]

SLEEPWALKING AND DREAMING

Before 1963, sleepwalking was thought to be dream enactment occurring out of REM sleep. However, sleep laboratory studies showed sleepwalking to be caused by partial arousals from deep (SWS) sleep. Nevertheless, the role of dreamlike mentation in sleepwalking episodes remains undefined and hypothetical. The occurrence of sleepwalking-related dreamlike mentation has been proposed as being reflective of mental processes that may occur during SWS.[34] However, it has also been argued that in sleepwalking episodes arising out of SWS, it is very unlikely that visual imagery or perception of narrative characteristic of REM dreams, or even vague ruminations characteristic of light non-REM sleep, could be present. It is hypothesized that SWS is not compatible with normal desynchronized cortical function. It can be hypothesized that in those with dreamlike experiences in the context of a non-REM arousal such as sleepwalking, these "dreams" may arise some time later after arousal onset. These dreamlike images or mentation may actually represent a confabulated cognitive correlate of an emotional state (such as fight or fright) generated subcortically, perhaps by the amygdala. This confabulation might be modified according to environmental stimuli seen or heard by the subject during the arousal. For example, the dreamlike experience of pets being in the bedroom or a partner being interpreted as an assailant or willing sexual partner may be incorporated into the image. The components of the "dream" thus generated may further psychically propel the ambulation or other automatic activity, which is effectively occurring in a confused state whereby some parts of the brain have awoken but some parts remain in SWS. In other words the non-REM "dream" may actually be a mixture of reality and confabulation. However, there is no scientific evidence to substantiate this hypothesis.

A more appealing idea discussed in the recent literature is that sleepwalking and other non-REM parasomnias might arise from a dissociation of sleep and wakefulness occurring across different brain regions, with some parts of the brain, such as the occipital lobes, displaying features of wakefulness with other regions showing sleep (see the article by Mahowald and colleagues elsewhere in this issue). In one report an EEG recording during a prolonged parasomnia showed alpha rhythm consistent with wakefulness in posterior channels with simultaneous anterior and midline theta activity and vertex sharp activity, consistent with stage 2 non-REM sleep.[30] In another reported case of a recorded episode of night terror with simultaneous EEG and cerebral SPECT scanning, there was increased activity in the posterior cingulate cortex whereas large areas of frontal and parietal association cortices remained deactivated.[31]

DIFFERENTIAL DIAGNOSIS

It is common for a sleep specialist to be asked for a clinical opinion on a patient presenting with nocturnal wandering. The key to narrowing down the diagnostic possibilities is knowledge of the differential diagnoses, and the formulation of a system by a detailed history-taking process supported by detailed PSG and EEG. An early case series comprised a group of young adults without a previous history of epilepsy presenting with episodic nocturnal wanderings. These wanderings were characterized by stereotyped frequent attacks of screaming, ambulation, and complex automatisms, including semipurposeful violent behavior. Four of the patients were found to have epileptiform activity. Anticonvulsant therapy reduced or eliminated the attacks in these 4 patients.[81] The exact cause of this behavior was undetermined in the others. A qualitative analysis of behavior patterns and ictal EEG was undertaken in one study of subjects with either parasomnia or nocturnal frontal lobe epilepsy (NFLE).[30] The investigators found that those with parasomnia had particular clinical features when compared with the NFLE group. These clinical features included interactive behavior, failure to wake after the event, and indistinct offset. Eighty-two percent of the seizure activity took place in non-REM stage 1 or 2 sleep, whereas 100% of parasomnia events in this group took place during SWS. There were 3 behavioral patterns seen in those with parasomnia: arousal behavior in 92%, nonagitated motor behavior in 72%, and distressed emotional behavior in 51%. The investigators concluded that sleepwalking, confusional arousals,

and night terrors form a hierarchical continuum rather than distinct entities.

In 100 consecutive adults attending a sleep disorders clinic with repeated nocturnal injury, PSG studies identified night terrors/sleepwalking in 54, RBD in 36, dissociative disorders in 7, nocturnal seizures in 2, and OSA in 1.[44] In another case series of 41 subjects between the age of 12 and 63 years presenting with nocturnal wanderings including violent behavior in their sleep, who underwent detailed PSG, and wake and sleep EEG including ambulatory EEG at home, temporal lobe abnormalities were seen particularly in those presenting with violent sleep behavior.[48] Males made up the majority of this group.

In a case series of 100 consecutive patients with NFLE,[82] the investigators found 3 non-REM–related subtypes of seizures: (1) paroxysmal arousals characterized by brief and sudden recurrent motor paroxysmal behavior; (2) nocturnal paroxysmal dystonia, and motor attacks with complex dystonic-dyskinetic features; and (3) episodic nocturnal wanderings, stereotyped and "agitated" sleepwalking. There was a family history of parasomnia in 39% of the group. Others have therefore concluded that patients presenting with episodic nocturnal wanderings, with a family history of sleepwalking, should still have detailed EEG recordings to rule out NFLE.[83] As PSG recordings may not pick up and capture complex episodes in a sleep laboratory, audio-video recordings at home may be considered.[84] Postictal confusion must also be differentiated from the confusional state related to a sleepwalking awakening.[85] However, in practice there may well be an overlap, in that seizures may cause arousals that lead to sleepwalking or confusional arousals. In fact frontal lobe seizures are considered to be often devoid of a surface EEG correlate, and patients with these seizures also display non-REM parasomnia-like phenomena.[82] It can therefore be very difficult to be sure what one is dealing with, and research that has sought to distinguish frontal seizures from non-REM parasomnia on the basis of generally accepted diagnostic features[30] may in fact promote a circular argument of diagnostic uncertainty.

DRUG-INDUCED SLEEPWALKING

There have been several case reports of medication, particularly those used commonly in psychiatric clinics, which purportedly induce sleepwalking. In a case series of 389 patients using lithium (the majority had bipolar affective disorder), 27 (6.9%) patients presented with sleepwalking behavior closely related to the onset of treatment with lithium alone or in combination with other psychotropic drugs.[86] Of this lithium group 45 patients suffered from sleepwalking as a child, and 12 had their sleepwalking reactivated by psychiatric medication. However, it has been suggested that "sleepwalking" in this group of heavily medicated patients may actually represent the effects of significant central nervous system (CNS) depression and not typical sleepwalking.[36] There have been numerous case reports of complex behaviors in sleep related to benzodiazepines and other drugs that act at the γ-aminobutyric acid (GABA) receptor, such as zolpidem,[87–90] zaleplon,[91] and zopiclone.[92] In a case series of 125 patients attending a psychiatric clinic who were taking zolpidem, 19 subjects (15%) had features of complex sleep-related behaviors such as sleepwalking and SRE after commencing this drug. In this group it was more common in younger females taking a higher dose (>10 mg).[93] The exact mechanism is unclear, but may be related to the enhancement of GABA activity at a receptor level that may also enhance the amnesic features.[94] Stopping the medications or reducing the dose is recommended. Due to the millions of prescriptions of benzodiazepines that are provided around the world, particularly zolpidem and zopiclone, issues of driving under the influence (DUI)-related police stops, arrests, and accidents resulting from this type of medication have been recently highlighted (see the article by Pressman elsewhere in this issue).[95] Many driving episodes attributed to sleep driving were instead determined to be more likely secondary to misuse and abuse of the sedative hypnotic drugs. Such drivers should not be confused with drivers who may be sleepwalking (although such cases are very rare). The symptoms of drug-related CNS depression are not identical to the symptoms or behaviors of a sleepwalker. The individual who misuses or abuses sedatives or hypnotics and experiences CNS depression may demonstrate cognitive functions at low levels. These individuals may still be able to understand and respond to questions, whereas sleepwalkers are completely unable to understand or interact with police. Sleepwalkers are able to stand and walk unaided, whereas those under the influence of sedatives or hypnotics will have difficulty standing unaided or maintaining balance It can be hypothesized that the sedative effects may generally suppress arousals, making them less frequent, but that if arousals do break through, then the sedative effect may suppress or delay full arousal, which may more likely result in the prolongation of confusion and hence possibly increase the duration of the episodes.

Other psychiatric drugs to induce sleepwalking that have been reported include amitryptyline,[96] olanzapine,[97–99] paroxetine,[100] risperidone,[101] quetiapine,[102] and mirtazepine.[103]

TREATMENT OF SLEEPWALKING

A recent review has highlighted the lack of adequately powered randomized controlled trials (RCTs) for the treatment (both pharmacologic and psychological) of sleepwalking.[104] There have been very few RCTs assessing interventions in comparison with placebo in sleepwalking. In a single, blinded prospective trial comparison of 10 mg diazepam in a small number of sleepwalkers (N = 5), there were inconsistent results in the alleviation of sleepwalking.[105] In a case cohort study of 170 adult referrals for disrupted nocturnal sleep treated with nightly benzodiazepines (of which 69 had features of sleepwalking and night terrors, 52 had RBD, and 25 had severe insomnia),[106] clonazepam was the most commonly used benzodiazepine (in 136 patients), with a mean initial dose of 0.77 mg and a mean final dose of 1.1 mg. The next most commonly used drug was alprazolam. Clonazepam was found to be effective in producing a complete or substantial control of the sleep disorders with a low risk of dosage tolerance, adverse effects, or dependency. In another case cohort study of 100 consecutive adults attending a sleep disorders clinic with a mixture of diagnoses including night terrors/sleepwalking in 54 and RBD in 36, clonazepam controlled the symptoms in 51 of the 61 patients.[44]

There are very few data on the usage of nonbenzodiazepines in sleepwalkers. The most commonly used nonbenzodiazepine drugs are antidepressants, particularly tricyclic antidepressants and serotonin-selective reuptake inhibitors.[107] These drugs may occasionally precipitate sleepwalking. There is a case report of the successful use of topiramate in a patient with sleepwalking, SRE, and PTSD.[108] A further retrospective survey of 30 cases of SRE disorder treated with topiramate (mean dose 135 mg and range 25–300 mg) over a mean period of 11.6 months found a positive response in 68%, with 28% losing more than 10% of their body weight.[109] However, 41% of patients discontinued topiramate after an average of 12 months because of intolerability. Further double-blind studies are warranted with this particular drug. Further reviews on nighttime eating disorders are available elsewhere.[110]

Treatment of comorbid sleep disorders has been described elsewhere in this article, but the literature does point to the assessment of possible coexistence of other sleep conditions, such as OSA and periodic limb movements, as part of the generalized workup in assessing and treating a sleepwalker.

The role of psychological therapy remains undetermined, with one small study producing a possible improvement in symptoms by hypnotherapy[111] and another study of the effect of hypnosis finding a 74% success rate in a group of 27 adult sleepwalkers and sleep terror sufferers.[112] Further 5-year follow-up in this group showed a 40% symptom-free prevalence after 5 years.[113] Other behavioral therapy that has been assessed in the treatment of sleepwalking, particularly in children, has been schedule awakening, whereby parents awake their children several hours after they go to bed and just before the typical time of a sleepwalking episode. One study in 3 children showed sustained treatment effects after 6 months.[114] However, there has been limited assessment of the efficacy of such therapies, and further research is needed to validate these methods.[115]

Better evidence is therefore necessary to support treatment decisions in sleepwalking, including adequately powered controlled trials, particularly to assess drug tolerance and side effects of benzodiazepine-related medications and the development of other nonbenzodiazepine drugs. Without such evidence, issues will remain regarding the prescription of such therapies as being off-label.[116]

SUMMARY

Sleepwalking is not a rare condition and most commonly occurs in children. Epidemiologic data have shown that the prevalence declines with age. There has been an increasing interest in the genetic basis of sleepwalking, although the role of genetic inheritance in predetermining risk remains undetermined but of great interest. Clinical features vary from individual to individual, and even vary as the individual gets older. Sleepwalking is not associated with higher cognitive behavior. Memory, planning, and social interaction are generally absent. Sleepwalking may be related to eating behavior during sleep, with the concomitant risk of excessive weight gain for many. Sleepwalkers have a predisposition (genetic) and several potential triggers to induce sleepwalking, particularly factors that would fragment sleep and cause arousals. Studies have shown that leg movements during sleep and sleep-disordered breathing may be potential triggers, and these factors need to be assessed by the sleep specialist. Violent and sexual behavior may occur during sleepwalking and, as a result, sleep specialists are being asked more and more to provide expert opinions to the courts on this matter. Knowledge of the published data and an understanding of the science of sleepwalking are critical for those sleep specialists who undertake legal expert witness activity for the courts. The exact role of SWS in sleepwalkers remains undetermined, and further research is necessary to characterize the role of abnormal SWS, particularly in response to sleep deprivation, and to assess the role of arousals in triggering sleepwalking episodes. The sleep specialist should be aware of the differential diagnoses of sleepwalking, particularly epilepsy, dissociative disorders, and other parasomnias, particularly RBD. The role of sleep deprivation, PSG, and external triggering using arousals needs further research and validation. There have been several drugs implicated in the induction of sleepwalking in numerous case reports. The most common drugs reported are GABA receptor agonists such as zolpidem and zopiclone. However, the optimal treatment of sleepwalking is undetermined by virtue of the lack of adequately powered RCTs. Clonazepam is the most commonly reported in the literature to show effectiveness, but only in the form of case cohort data. Sleepwalking is a fascinating facet of nature that is much more common than is generally thought. The current research on sleepwalking has increased exponentially in recent years, and continuing research in its diagnosis, neurophysiology, and treatment will further inform the sleep specialist.

REFERENCES

1. Broughton RJ. Sleep disorders: disorders of arousal? Enuresis, somnambulism, and nightmares occur in confusional states of arousal, not in "dreaming sleep". Science 1968;159:1070–8.
2. Kavey NB, Whyte J, Resor SR Jr, et al. Somnambulism in adults. Neurology 1990;40:749–52.
3. Blatt I, Peled R, Gadoth N, et al. The value of sleep recording in evaluating somnambulism in young adults. Electroencephalogr Clin Neurophysiol 1991;78:407–12.
4. Zadra A, Pilon M, Joncas S, et al. Analysis of post-arousal EEG activity during somnambulistic episodes. J Sleep Res 2004;13:279–84.
5. Schenck CH, Pareja JA, Patterson AL, et al. Analysis of polysomnographic events surrounding 252 slow-wave sleep arousals in thirty-eight adults with injurious sleepwalking and sleep terrors. J Clin Neurophysiol 1998;15:159–66.

6. Espa F, Ondze B, Deglise P, et al. Sleep architecture, slow wave activity, and sleep spindles in adult patients with sleepwalking and sleep terrors. Clin Neurophysiol 2000;111:929–39.

7. Gaudreau H, Joncas S, Zadra A, et al. Dynamics of slow-wave activity during the NREM sleep of sleepwalkers and control subjects. Sleep 2000;23:755–60.

8. Guilleminault C, Poyares D, Aftab FA, et al. Sleep and wakefulness in somnambulism: a spectral analysis study. J Psychosom Res 2001;51:411–6.

9. Pilon M, Zadra A, Joncas S, et al. Hypersynchronous delta waves and somnambulism: brain topography and effect of sleep deprivation. Sleep 2006; 29:77–84.

10. Pressman MR. Hypersynchronous delta sleep EEG activity and sudden arousals from slow-wave sleep in adults without a history of parasomnias: clinical and forensic implications. Sleep 2004;27:706–10.

11. Guilleminault C, Lee JH, Chan A, et al. Non-REM-sleep instability in recurrent sleepwalking in pre-pubertal children. Sleep Med 2005;6:515–21.

12. Guilleminault C, Kirisoglu C, da Rosa AC, et al. Sleepwalking, a disorder of NREM sleep instability. Sleep Med 2006;7:163–70.

13. Jaar O, Pilon M, Carrier J, et al. Analysis of slow-wave activity and slow-wave oscillations prior to somnambulism. Sleep 2010;33:1511–6.

14. Pressman MR. Why has sleepwalking research been "sleepwalking"? Neurology 2008;70:2274–5.

15. Kotagal S. Parasomnias of childhood. Curr Opin Pediatr 2008;20:659–65.

16. Liu X, Ma Y, Wang Y, et al. Brief report: an epidemiologic survey of the prevalence of sleep disorders among children 2 to 12 years old in Beijing, China. Pediatrics 2005;115:266–8.

17. Petit D, Touchette E, Tremblay RE, et al. Dyssomnias and parasomnias in early childhood. Pediatrics 2007;119:e1016–25.

18. Ohayon MM, Guilleminault C, Priest RG. Night terrors, sleepwalking, and confusional arousals in the general population: their frequency and relationship to other sleep and mental disorders. J Clin Psychiatry 1999;60:268–76.

19. Santos-Silva R, Bittencourt LR, Pires ML, et al. Increasing trends of sleep complaints in the city of Sao Paulo, Brazil. Sleep Med 2010;11:520–4.

20. Eitner S, Urschitz MS, Guenther A, et al. Sleep problems and daytime somnolence in a German population-based sample of snoring school-aged children. J Sleep Res 2007;16:96–101.

21. Bixler EO, Kales A, Soldatos CR, et al. Prevalence of sleep disorders in the Los Angeles metropolitan area. Am J Psychiatry 1979;136:1257–62.

22. Hublin C, Kaprio J, Partinen M, et al. Prevalence and genetics of sleepwalking: a population-based twin study. Neurology 1997;48:177–81.

23. Laberge L, Tremblay RE, Vitaro F, et al. Development of parasomnias from childhood to early adolescence. Pediatrics 2000;106:67–74.

24. Cao M, Guilleminault C. Families with sleepwalking. Sleep Med 2010;11:726–34.

25. Licis AK, Desruisseau DM, Yamada KA, et al. Novel genetic findings in an extended family pedigree with sleepwalking. Neurology 2011;76:49–52.

26. Dogu O, Pressman MR. Identification of sleepwalking gene(s): not yet, but soon? Neurology 2011;76: 12–3.

27. Schenck CH, Boyd JL, Mahowald MW. A parasomnia overlap disorder involving sleepwalking, sleep terrors, and REM sleep behavior disorder in 33 polysomnographically confirmed cases. Sleep 1997;20:972–81.

28. Schenck CH, Mahowald MW. Two cases of premenstrual sleep terrors and injurious sleepwalking. J Psychosom Obstet Gynaecol 1995;16: 79–84.

29. Cartwright R. Re: Pressman, M. Factors that predispose, prime and precipitate NREM parasomnias in adults: clinical and forensic implications. Sleep Med Rev 2007;11:5–30. Sleep Med Rev 2007;11:327–9.

30. Derry CP, Harvey AS, Walker MC, et al. NREM arousal parasomnias and their distinction from nocturnal frontal lobe epilepsy: a video EEG analysis. Sleep 2009;32:1637–44.

31. Bassetti C, Vella S, Donati F, et al. SPECT during sleepwalking. Lancet 2000;356:484–5.

32. Montplaisir J, Petit D, Pilon M, et al. Does sleepwalking impair daytime vigilance? J Clin Sleep Med 2011;7:219.

33. Mehlenbeck R, Spirito A, Owens J, et al. The clinical presentation of childhood partial arousal parasomnias. Sleep Med 2000;1:307–12.

34. Oudiette D, Leu S, Pottier M, et al. Dreamlike mentations during sleepwalking and sleep terrors in adults. Sleep 2009;32:1621–7.

35. Hartman D, Crisp AH, Sedgwick P, et al. Is there a dissociative process in sleepwalking and night terrors? Postgrad Med J 2001;77:244–9.

36. Pressman MR. Factors that predispose, prime and precipitate NREM parasomnias in adults: clinical and forensic implications. Sleep Med Rev 2007; 11:5–30.

37. Joncas S, Zadra A, Paquet J, et al. The value of sleep deprivation as a diagnostic tool in adult sleepwalkers. Neurology 2002;58:936–40.

38. Pilon M, Montplaisir J, Zadra A. Precipitating factors of somnambulism: impact of sleep deprivation and forced arousals. Neurology 2008;70: 2284–90.

39. Zadra A, Pilon M, Montplaisir J. Polysomnographic diagnosis of sleepwalking: effects of sleep deprivation. Ann Neurol 2008;63:513–9.

40. Pressman MR, Mahowald MW, Schenck CH, et al. Alcohol-induced sleepwalking or confusional arousal as a defense to criminal behavior: a review of scientific evidence, methods and forensic considerations. J Sleep Res 2007;16:198–212.

41. Schenck CH, Mahowald MW. An analysis of a recent criminal trial involving sexual misconduct with a child, alcohol abuse and a successful sleepwalking defence: arguments supporting two proposed new forensic categories. Med Sci Law 1998;38:147–52.

42. Hedman C, Pohjasvaara T, Tolonen U, et al. Parasomnias decline during pregnancy. Acta Neurol Scand 2002;105:209–14.

43. Ipsiroglu OS, Fatemi A, Werner I, et al. Self-reported organic and nonorganic sleep problems in schoolchildren aged 11 to 15 years in Vienna. J Adolesc Health 2002;31:436–42.

44. Schenck CH, Milner DM, Hurwitz TD, et al. A polysomnographic and clinical report on sleep-related injury in 100 adult patients. Am J Psychiatry 1989;146:1166–73.

45. Guilleminault C, Leger D, Philip P, et al. Nocturnal wandering and violence: review of a sleep clinic population. J Forensic Sci 1998;43:158–63.

46. Shatkin JP, Feinfield K, Strober M. The misinterpretation of a non-REM sleep parasomnia as suicidal behavior in an adolescent. Sleep Breath 2002;6:175–9.

47. Mahowald MW, Schenck CH, Goldner M, et al. Parasomnia pseudo-suicide. J Forensic Sci 2003;48:1158–62.

48. Guilleminault C, Moscovitch A, Leger D. Forensic sleep medicine: nocturnal wandering and violence. Sleep 1995;18:740–8.

49. Mahowald MW, Schenck CH, Cramer-Bornemann MA. Sleep-related violence. Curr Neurol Neurosci Rep 2005;5:153–8.

50. Pressman MR. Disorders of arousal from sleep and violent behavior: the role of physical contact and proximity. Sleep 2007;30:1039–47.

51. Broughton R, Billings R, Cartwright R, et al. Homicidal somnambulism: a case report. Sleep 1994;17:253–64.

52. Moldofsky H, Gilbert R, Lue FA, et al. Sleep-related violence. Sleep 1995;18:731–9.

53. Schenck CH, Mahowald MW. A polysomnographically documented case of adult somnambulism with long-distance automobile driving and frequent nocturnal violence: parasomnia with continuing danger as a noninsane automatism? Sleep 1995;18:765–72.

54. Mahowald MW, Schenck CH. Parasomnias: sleepwalking and the law. Sleep Med Rev 2000;4:321–39.

55. Grunstein R. Guest editorial: was O. J. sleepwalking? Sleep Med Rev 2000;4:319–20.

56. Pressman MR, Schenck CH, Mahowald MW, et al. Sleep science in the courtroom. J Forensic Leg Med 2007;14:108–11.

57. Mahowald MW, Schenck CH, Cramer-Bornemann M. Finally—sleep science for the courtroom. Sleep Med Rev 2007;11:1–3.

58. Pressman MR, Mahowald MW, Schenck CH, et al. Sleep-related automatism and the law. Med Sci Law 2009;49:139–43.

59. Shapiro CM, Trajanovic NN, Fedoroff JP. Sexsomnia—a new parasomnia? Can J Psychiatry 2003;48:311–7.

60. Buchanan A. Sleepwalking and indecent exposure. Med Sci Law 1991;31:38–40.

61. Bowden P. Sleepwalking and indecent exposure. Med Sci Law 1991;31:359.

62. Schenck CH, Arnulf I, Mahowald MW. Sleep and sex: what can go wrong? A review of the literature on sleep related disorders and abnormal sexual behaviors and experiences. Sleep 2007;30:683–702.

63. Guilleminault C, Palombini L, Pelayo R, et al. Sleepwalking and sleep terrors in prepubertal children: what triggers them? Pediatrics 2003;111:e17–25.

64. Espa F, Dauvilliers Y, Ondze B, et al. Arousal reactions in sleepwalking and night terrors in adults: the role of respiratory events. Sleep 2002;25:871–5.

65. Guilleminault C, Kirisoglu C, Bao G, et al. Adult chronic sleepwalking and its treatment based on polysomnography. Brain 2005;128:1062–9.

66. Alonso-Navarro H, Jimenez-Jimenez FJ. Restless legs syndrome associated with narcolepsy and somnambulism. Parkinsonism Relat Disord 2010;16:146–7.

67. Schenck CH, Hurwitz TD, Bundlie SR, et al. Sleep-related eating disorders: polysomnographic correlates of a heterogeneous syndrome distinct from daytime eating disorders. Sleep 1991;14:419–31.

68. Vetrugno R, Manconi M, Ferini-Strambi L, et al. Nocturnal eating: sleep-related eating disorder or night eating syndrome? A videopolysomnographic study. Sleep 2006;29:949–54.

69. Winkelman JW. Clinical and polysomnographic features of sleep-related eating disorder. J Clin Psychiatry 1998;59:14–9.

70. Crisp AH, Matthews BM, Oakey M, et al. Sleepwalking, night terrors, and consciousness. BMJ 1990;300:360–2.

71. Lam SP, Fong SY, Ho CK, et al. Parasomnia among psychiatric outpatients: a clinical, epidemiologic, cross-sectional study. J Clin Psychiatry 2008;69:1374–82.

72. Lam SP, Fong SY, Yu MW, et al. Sleepwalking in psychiatric patients: comparison of childhood and adult onset. Aust N Z J Psychiatry 2009;43:426–30.

73. Shang CY, Gau SS, Soong WT. Association between childhood sleep problems and perinatal

factors, parental mental distress and behavioral problems. J Sleep Res 2006;15:63–73.

74. Silvestri R, Gagliano A, Arico I, et al. Sleep disorders in children with attention-deficit/hyperactivity disorder (ADHD) recorded overnight by video-polysomnography. Sleep Med 2009;10:1132–8.

75. Gau SF, Soong WT. Psychiatric comorbidity of adolescents with sleep terrors or sleepwalking: a case-control study. Aust N Z J Psychiatry 1999; 33:734–9.

76. Merlino G, Piani A, Dolso P, et al. Sleep disorders in patients with end-stage renal disease undergoing dialysis therapy. Nephrol Dial Transplant 2006;21: 184–90.

77. Poryazova R, Waldvogel D, Bassetti CL. Sleepwalking in patients with Parkinson disease. Arch Neurol 2007;64:1524–7.

78. Oberholzer M, Poryazova R, Bassetti CL. Sleepwalking in Parkinson's disease: a questionnaire-based survey. J Neurol 2011;258(7):1261–7.

79. Mouzas O, Angelopoulos N, Papaliagka M, et al. Increased frequency of self-reported parasomnias in patients suffering from vitiligo. Eur J Dermatol 2008;18:165–8.

80. Merlino G, Piani A, Gigli GL, et al. Daytime sleepiness is associated with dementia and cognitive decline in older Italian adults: a population-based study. Sleep Med 2010;11:372–7.

81. Maselli RA, Rosenberg RS, Spire JP. Episodic nocturnal wanderings in non-epileptic young patients. Sleep 1988;11:156–61.

82. Provini F, Plazzi G, Tinuper P, et al. Nocturnal frontal lobe epilepsy. A clinical and polygraphic overview of 100 consecutive cases. Brain 1999;122(Pt 6): 1017–31.

83. Farid M, Kushida CA. Non-rapid eye movement parasomnias. Curr Treat Options Neurol 2004;6: 331–7.

84. Plazzi G, Vetrugno R, Provini F, et al. Sleepwalking and other ambulatory behaviours during sleep. Neurol Sci 2005;26(Suppl 3):s193–8.

85. Bazil CW. Effects of sleep on the postictal state. Epilepsy Behav 2010;19:146–50.

86. Landry P, Warnes H, Nielsen T, et al. Somnambulistic-like behaviour in patients attending a lithium clinic. Int Clin Psychopharmacol 1999;14:173–5.

87. Siddiqui F, Osuna E, Chokroverty S. Writing emails as part of sleepwalking after increase in Zolpidem. Sleep Med 2009;10:262–4.

88. Hoque R, Chesson AL Jr. Zolpidem-induced sleepwalking, sleep related eating disorder, and sleep-driving: fluorine-18-flourodeoxyglucose positron emission tomography analysis, and a literature review of other unexpected clinical effects of zolpidem. J Clin Sleep Med 2009;5:471–6.

89. Sattar SP, Ramaswamy S, Bhatia SC, et al. Somnambulism due to probable interaction of valproic acid and zolpidem. Ann Pharmacother 2003;37:1429–33.

90. Iruela LM. Zolpidem and sleepwalking. J Clin Psychopharmacol 1995;15:223.

91. Liskow B, Pikalov A. Zaleplon overdose associated with sleepwalking and complex behavior. J Am Acad Child Adolesc Psychiatry 2004;43:927–8.

92. Ferentinos P, Paparrigopoulos T. Zopiclone and sleepwalking. Int J Neuropsychopharmacol 2009; 12:141–2.

93. Hwang TJ, Ni HC, Chen HC, et al. Risk predictors for hypnosedative-related complex sleep behaviors: a retrospective, cross-sectional pilot study. J Clin Psychiatry 2010;71:1331–5.

94. Dolder CR, Nelson MH. Hypnosedative-induced complex behaviours: incidence, mechanisms and management. CNS Drugs 2008;22:1021–36.

95. Pressman MR. Sleep driving: sleepwalking variant or misuse of z-drugs? Sleep Med Rev 2011;15(5): 285–92.

96. Ferrandiz-Santos JA, Mataix-Sanjuan AL. Amitriptyline and somnambulism. Ann Pharmacother 2000; 34:1208.

97. Kolivakis TT, Margolese HC, Beauclair L, et al. Olanzapine-induced somnambulism. Am J Psychiatry 2001;158:1158.

98. Paquet V, Strul J, Servais L, et al. Sleep-related eating disorder induced by olanzapine. J Clin Psychiatry 2002;63:597.

99. Chiu YH, Chen CH, Shen WW. Somnambulism secondary to olanzapine treatment in one patient with bipolar disorder. Prog Neuropsychopharmacol Biol Psychiatry 2008;32:581–2.

100. Kawashima T, Yamada S. Paroxetine-induced somnambulism. J Clin Psychiatry 2003;64:483.

101. Lu ML, Shen WW. Sleep-related eating disorder induced by risperidone. J Clin Psychiatry 2004; 65:273–4.

102. Hafeez ZH, Kalinowski CM. Somnambulism induced by quetiapine: two case reports and a review of the literature. CNS Spectr 2007;12:910–2.

103. Yeh YW, Chen CH, Feng HM, et al. New onset somnambulism associated with different dosage of mirtazapine: a case report. Clin Neuropharmacol 2009;32:232–3.

104. Harris M, Grunstein RR. Treatments for somnambulism in adults: assessing the evidence. Sleep Med Rev 2009;13:295–7.

105. Reid WH, Haffke EA, Chu CC. Diazepam in intractable sleepwalking: a pilot study. Hillside J Clin Psychiatry 1984;6:49–55.

106. Schenck CH, Mahowald MW. Long-term, nightly benzodiazepine treatment of injurious parasomnias and other disorders of disrupted nocturnal sleep in 170 adults. Am J Med 1996;100:333–7.

107. Remulla A, Guilleminault C. Somnambulism (sleepwalking). Expert Opin Pharmacother 2004;5:2069–74.

108. Tucker P, Masters B, Nawar O. Topiramate in the treatment of comorbid night eating syndrome and PTSD: a case study. Eat Disord 2004;12: 75–8.

109. Winkelman JW. Efficacy and tolerability of open-label topiramate in the treatment of sleep-related eating disorder: a retrospective case series. J Clin Psychiatry 2006;67:1729–34.

110. Howell MJ, Schenck CH, Crow SJ. A review of night-time eating disorders. Sleep Med Rev 2009;13:23–34.

111. Reid WH, Ahmed I, Levie CA. Treatment of sleep-walking: a controlled study. Am J Psychother 1981;35:27–37.

112. Hurwitz TD, Mahowald MW, Schenck CH, et al. A retrospective outcome study and review of hypnosis as treatment of adults with sleepwalking and sleep terror. J Nerv Ment Dis 1991;179:228–33.

113. Hauri PJ, Silber MH, Boeve BF. The treatment of parasomnias with hypnosis: a 5-year follow-up study. J Clin Sleep Med 2007;3:369–73.

114. Frank NC, Spirito A, Stark L, et al. The use of scheduled awakenings to eliminate childhood sleepwalking. J Pediatr Psychol 1997;22:345–53.

115. Sadeh A. Cognitive-behavioral treatment for childhood sleep disorders. Clin Psychol Rev 2005;25: 612–28.

116. Gazarian M, Kelly M, McPhee JR, et al. Off-label use of medicines: consensus recommendations for evaluating appropriateness. Med J Aust 2006; 185:544–8.

Sleep Sex

Peter R. Buchanan, MD, FRACP[a,b,c,*]

KEYWORDS

• Sleep sex • Parasomnia • Forensics

Human sleep and sex are closely connected. Sexual activity during wake may proximally precede a major sleep period, be interspersed during wake episodes within a major sleep period, and may follow a major sleep period during (usually morning) wake. Sleep may provide the restorative quality that lends to participation in wake sexual activity, and sometimes provides a physiologic basis for opportunity via, for example, rapid eye movement (REM) sleep stage arousal phenomena that persist to wake. Sexual activity, at least in men, may promote entry into sleep, or alternatively lead to a state of hyper-arousal. Human sexual activity may also occur without close temporal proximity to sleep periods. In its substantive content, human sexual activity can potentially be polymorphously perverse, and the timing of human sexual activity can be unpredictably irregular or monotonously scheduled.

Human sexual activity is a complex and (usually) gratifying behavior that amalgamates volitional initiative psychoerotic components with behavioral, motor, and reflexive autonomic physiologic phenomena. In most circumstances, sleep also involves a volitional initiation conditioned by complex physiologic factors and followed by a highly organized and controlled expression of sleep behavior.

However, in some unusual circumstances, sleep and sex do not have a formal state-based separation. Sexual activity may arise and act out during sleep, or may apparently do so, and this phenomenon is the subject of this article.

DEFINITIONS AND NOSOLOGIES

The terms sleep sex, sleepsex, sexual behavior in sleep, sexsomnia, abnormal or atypical sexual behavior during sleep, and somnambulistic sexual behavior have been used interchangeably in the literature of this topic.[1–5] For simplicity, this article follows editorial lead and (except when quoting sources) uses the term sleep sex. This article does not further discuss other sexual phenomena that manifest during or from sleep, such as REM-related nocturnal penile tumescence,[6] painful penile erections,[7] nocturnal emissions, or hypersexuality syndromes that occur in wake or sleep-wake transition states (including Kleine-Levin syndrome[8]), sexual hallucinations as part of narcolepsy,[9] and so forth.

There are limited published data from which to review the subject of human sleep sex. Most, if not all, such data are from case reports, observational case series, and reviews. There is also some information from Internet Web-based surveys. In the forensic context, some data come from legal reports. Thus the data sources for any review of sleep sex emanate from the lower reaches of the evidence base pyramid.

Sleep sex is mentioned in the International Classification of Sleep Disorders (ICSD) second edition 2005, as a variant of the non-REM parasomnias, confusional arousal, and sleepwalking.[10] Quoting from ICSD second edition 2005:

Sleep related abnormal sexual behaviors can be primarily classified as confusional

---

The author has nothing to disclose that is relevant to this article.

[a] Sleep and Circadian Research Group, NHMRC Centre for Integrated Research and Understanding of Sleep (CIRUS), Woolcock Institute of Medical Research, PO Box M77, Missenden Road, NSW 2050, Australia
[b] Department of Respiratory Medicine, Liverpool Hospital, Elizabeth Street, Liverpool, NSW 2170, Australia
[c] Sleep Disorders Service, Suite 806, St Vincent's Clinic, 438 Victoria Street, Darlinghurst, Sydney, NSW 2010, Australia
* Sleep and Circadian Research Group, NHMRC Centre for Integrated Research and Understanding of Sleep (CIRUS), Woolcock Institute of Medical Research, PO Box M77, Missenden Road, NSW 2050, Australia.
E-mail address: pbuchanan@woolcock.org.au

Sleep Med Clin 6 (2011) 417–428
doi:10.1016/j.jsmc.2011.08.006

arousals. 'Atypical sexual behavior during sleep', 'sexsomnia' and 'sleepsex' comprise a recently described parasomnia that often has major interpersonal and clinical consequences. These sleep related abnormal sexual behaviors usually occur during confusional arousals but can also occur with sleepwalking. The set of abnormal sexual behaviors during disordered arousals includes prolonged or violent masturbation, sexual molestation and assaults (of minors and adults), initiation of sexual intercourse irrespective of the menstrual status of the bed partner (unlike during waking intercourse for those individuals), and loud (sexual) vocalizations during sleep – followed by morning amnesia. The preponderance of patients has conditions that have been diagnosed as a NREM sleep parasomnia, either confusional arousals alone or together with sleepwalking (and at times with sleep-related driving of an automobile or with SRED).

The ICSD is a working platform of sleep medicine disorders nosology, with significant elements defined by a combination of best currently available scientific evidence and structured consensual expert opinion. This qualification is particularly relevant to the topic of sleep sex.

The psychiatric coding manual the *Diagnostic and Statistical Manual of Mental Disorders, Fourth Edition, Text Revision* (DSM-IV-TR)[11] does not specifically mention sleep sex as a diagnostic consideration under parasomnias. The parasomnias classification of the DSM-IV-TR is peremptory and reflective of an earlier point of knowledge, and whether sleep sex will be recognized in DSM-V remains to be seen. The International Classification of Diseases-10, under Mental and Behavioral Disorders, lists nonorganic sleep disorders (F51) to include parasomnias like sleepwalking, night terrors, and other nonorganic sleep disorders, specified and unspecified, but sleep sex is not specifically listed.[12] Most practicing sleep physicians and others interested in this area defer to ICSD second edition 2005 as the nosologic reference of first choice on this topic.

HISTORICAL ASPECTS OF SLEEP SEX REPORTING

It is probable that sleep sex has occurred across human history but, apart from likely scenarios described in (English) literature (eg, Thomas Hardy's 1891 novel *Tess of the D'Urbervilles*), without written scientific record until recent times, that prospect is largely obscured by time. There

are scattered more recent reports in medicolegal tracts[13] and psychiatric journals[14] but the modern age of published reporting on sleep sex began only in the 1980s.

Hartman[15] reported a middle-aged man with a history of sleepwalking and night terrors who, with alcohol as a putative factor, allegedly during sleep sexually assaulted his daughters. Wong[16] described a case of masturbation during sleep in a man beset by increased life stresses and prone to sleeptalking and sleep terrors. Hurwitz and colleagues[17] described a young male shift worker who was documented as having obstructive sleep apnea (OSA) on polysomnography (PSG) and who allegedly during sleep sexually assaulted a child; another case in the same abstract described a man with history of sleepwalking, sleep terror, and enuresis, with alcohol and another drug as putative cofactors, allegedly during sleep sexually assaulting his daughter. Buchanan[18] described a case of indecent exposure occurring during apparent sleep in a young man with a history of sleepwalking and in a context of stress, alcohol use, and sleep deprivation. Most of these cases from the 1980s and early 1990s had medicolegal ramifications and, with 1 exception, did not undergo standard tests of sleep disorders, such as PSG, and all were men.

CLINICAL CASE SERIES OF SLEEP SEX

More recent published cases of sleep sex also predominantly involve men, and often involve medicolegal considerations, and were more likely to be investigated with sleep studies. However, there have been some case series or case reports published in the last 20 years that inform current concepts of sleep sex. It is useful to review these in approximately chronologic sequence.

Guilleminault and colleagues[5] described a series of 11 patients referred to a Sleep Disorders Clinic because of atypical sexual behavior, 7 of whom were men. Sexual behavior ranged from sexualized moaning, through masturbation, to sexual assault involving attempted and actual fondling and sexual intercourse. Seven of the 11 had a personal history consistent with non-REM or other parasomnia (sleepwalking, sleep terrors, enuresis). Three other patients had attributable REM sleep behavior disorder, and 1 was diagnosed with complex partial seizure disorder. Psychiatric diagnoses were comorbid features in 7 of 11 patients (depression, obsessive compulsive personality trait, anxiety disorder). Unwanted sleep sex behavior was reported as controlled in 10 of 11 patients by the use of psychotropic medication in 8 (mostly clonazepam), continuous positive airway pressure (CPAP) and psycho-therapy in 1 case, and antiepileptic therapy in 1.

Shapiro and colleagues[3] presented a descriptive case series of 11 patients referred to a tertiary sleep clinic who manifested various sexual behaviors during sleep. The described behaviors included actual or attempted orogenital sex (cunnilingus) and sexual intercourse, sexual/genital touching, digital vaginal penetration, and masturbation. The 2 women in this series both masturbated as their sleep sex manifestation, 5 of the 11 cases had attendant medicolegal issues (although those issues were said to be related to sleep sex only in 3), and 1 man had comorbid OSA, which, when successfully treated with CPAP, led to remission of the sleep sex activity. PSG was performed in 9 of the 11 cases and reported to display features consistent with non-REM parasomnia (including the case with comorbid OSA). The attributable PSG features reported in these cases included abrupt arousals from slow wave sleep (SWS), redistribution of SWS across the whole sleep period, or nonspecified supportive features. However, there was no video-PSG documentation of any behavioral features of sleep sex in any case. The only exception being where video recording was performed on a sleeping couple and the nonpatient wife initiated and performed sexual activity with the engaged and then participating patient/husband while he was recorded to be drifting between stage 1 sleep and wakefulness, and he denied recall of such activity next morning. This event might be construed as an example of passive sleep sex, as may also the protagonist Tess in Hardy's fictional account (also see later discussion).

Della Marca and colleagues[19] described a triplet of sleep sex cases, attributable to OSA in 1 case, non-REM parasomnia in the second, and to REM sleep behavior disorder (RBD) in the third. Bejot and colleagues[20] describe 2 female cases of abnormal sexual behavior during sleep that the investigators attributed to sexsomnia variant of non-REM parasomnia. Although the described behavior fits the phenomenology of sleep sex behaviors, and 1 of the cases had a preceding history of sleepwalking, significant psychiatric comorbidity was present in both cases, although no dissociative disorder was documented by psychiatric assessment in either case. PSG showed abrupt arousals from SWS, but no overt sexual behavior. Both patients appeared to respond to selective serotonin reuptake inhibitor (SSRI) antidepressant pharmacotherapy, albeit slowly, and the second case was associated with recovery from major depressive disorder. A recent abstract described sleep sex in 2 generations (father and

son) of a family[21]; the clinical descriptions accord with non-REM parasomnia sleep sex and responded satisfactorily in both cases to clonazepam therapy.

WEB-BASED AND OTHER DATA ON SLEEP SEX

Trajanovic and colleagues[4] (also Mangan and Reips[22]) analyzed the results of a 28-item survey posted on an Internet Web site and reported 219 validated responses. Nearly one-third were women, episodes of sleep sex were multiple, and nearly half reported other parasomnias. Reported behaviors included sexualized movements and vocalizations, fondling, masturbation, and intercourse. A small number (15 of 219, of which 13 were men) were reported as having legal repercussions because of the sleep sex behaviors. Because of the nature of the selection process of this Internet Web-based survey, and the lack of a corroborative clinical assessment, a true estimate of the community prevalence of sleep sex cannot be established from this study.

Another study reported a 2% prevalence of sleep-related violence from a surveyed population[23] but did not subattribute any such instances as being related to sleep sex behavior. In a retrospective survey of the charts of 832 patients at a sleep disorders referral clinic, and using a patient questionnaire response, those who claimed to have initiated sexual activity with a bed partner while asleep were considered to have symptoms of sexomnia: 63/832 (7.6%) gave a positive response (men 11.0%, women 4.0%).[24] These figures reflect a selection bias to the clinic and identified cases were not otherwise validated independently from the questionnaire, so the derived figures cannot reliably be imputed to a general population prevalence.

Taking into account the limited numbers of cases available in published data, and the impression from clinical practice, sleep sex is not a common behavior presenting to physicians/health care providers. Adequate data from which to estimate true community prevalence are lacking.

PUBLISHED REVIEWS OF SLEEP SEX

Schenck and colleagues[8] provide a review of a broad range of sleep-related abnormal sexual behaviors and experiences including, but not limited to, sleep sex behavior associated with a diagnosis of non-REM parasomnia, and with epilepsy. The bulk of their cases reviewed in these latter categories come from the published case series of Guilleminault and colleagues[5] and

Shapiro and colleagues,[3] reviewed earlier, as well as a few additional cases drawn from the literature.

Their analysis of 31 cases of parasomnia-related sleep sex included 28 disorders of arousal (confusional arousals in 26, sleepwalking in 2, OSA comorbid in 4) and 3 cases of RBD. Duration of sleep sex was known/applicable in only 8 patients with a mean of 9.6 years (standard deviation ±6.1), with another 8 having had only 1 reported episode at time of publication. Of these 8 once-only cases, it is unclear how many were associated with legal ramifications, although, of the whole collected series of 31 cases, 11 (35%) were so associated. In the article by Guilleminault and colleagues,[5] the investigators note that "the only 2 cases seen at the first observation of abnormal sexual behavior during sleep were those involving police intervention." Male/female ratio was 4:1 in this collated sleep sex parasomnia–specific group.

Schenck and colleagues[8] tentatively identified some contrasting findings in the small group (n = 7) of accumulated epilepsy-related sleep sex cases. Proportionally more female cases were represented (43%). Presumably ictal-exclusive phenomena such as ictal orgasm were reported. The majority had some recall (next day) of the sleep sex behavior. Only a minority of these reported epilepsy-related sleep sex cases had undergone PSG or sleep electroencephalography (EEG).

Andersen and colleagues[25] tabulated in toto the historical case series, an additional (n = 7) series from Fenwick[26] that did not undergo any PSG evaluation, the Shapiro and colleagues[3] series and the Guilleminault and colleagues[5] series, and a few other case reports. This tabulation includes 3 cases of naked sleepwalking without sexual elements and 2 cases of what might be termed passive sexual intercourse in sleep perpetrated on a sleeping female by a wake person: it is debatable whether these cases should be considered as versions of sleep sex. Thirty-one of these 39 cases were men (79%), 24 of the 39 had a history of sleepwalking (and 1 of confusional arousal), thus 64% of this tabulated group had evidence by history of preexisting other non-REM parasomnia, 6 had a history of sleep talking only, and 1 subject was described as having excessive leg movements (during dreams). When discussing the diagnostic approach in difficult cases, Andersen and colleagues[25] mention provoking measures to bring out sleepwalking (and, by implication, sleepwalking variant activity such as sleep sex) during video-PSG monitoring, and include prior sleep deprivation and arousal (presumably auditory) during SWS, for both of which approaches there are published supportive data at least for non–sleep sex parasomnia behaviors,[27,28] and using

alcohol before bedtime; this latter approach for which there are no good, supportive, published data in this context.

Trajanovic and Shapiro[29] used the same data set of cases when presenting their review of sexsomnia. Again, the emphasis was on the association between sleep sex behavior and a recognizable non-REM parasomnia background. They also emphasized the differential diagnosis of sleep sex (suspected sexsomnia) to include non-REM parasomnias, RBD, seizure disorders, dissociative states, and malingering.

CLINICAL SYNTHESIS AND CAUSES

In published data, the included sexual behaviors within the sleep sex set have ranged across a variety of human sexual behaviors also encountered in wake subjects. These behaviors include sexual or sexualized moaning and overt vocalization (sex talk, dirty talk), sexualized body movements (eg, pelvic thrusting), masturbation, genital fondling, orogenital sex (fellatio, cunnilingus), digital vaginal/anal penetration, and heterosexual and homosexual full intercourse (**Box 1**). Individuals may engage in a sexual repertoire during sleep sex that differs from their preferences when engaging in sex activity during wake. The affective component of sexual behaviors may also differ between wake and sleep, the out-of-wake character being more enthusiastic, carefree, or experimental (although this is a subjective element perceived and reported by the bed/sexual partner).

From an analytical-clinical perspective, sleep sex might best be regarded as a syndrome of sleep-related sexual behaviors driven by various specific causes (**Box 2**). The syndrome itself comprises a set of sexual behaviors that occur during or from sleep, or are perceived as occurring

---

Box 1
Phenomenology of sleep sex

- Sexual or sexualized moaning, overt sexual vocalization (sex talk, dirty talk)
- Sexualized body movements (eg, pelvic thrusting)
- Masturbation
- Genital fondling
- Orogenital sex (fellatio, cunnilingus)
- Digital vaginal/anal penetration
- Heterosexual and homosexual full intercourse

> **Box 2**
> **Causes of sleep sex**
>
> - Non-REM parasomnia sleepwalking and confusional arousal
> - Sleep disordered breathing
> - RBD
> - Sleep epilepsy
> - Sleep-related dissociative disorders
> - Medication
> - Malingering

during a sleep period. Because most sleep episodes are nocturnal, this means that this behavior is usually nocturnal, although there is no inherent reason why sleep sex may not occur in a daytime sleep setting. That such sleep sex behavior has or has not occurred in or from sleep may also be a matter of further deliberation once an individual has presented for an initial assessment of putative sleep sex.

The most common cause linked with sleep sex in reported cases has been the non-REM parasomnias, or disorders of arousal. Combining the modern series of case reports of Guilleminault and colleagues[5] and Shapiro and colleagues,[3] and the 3 and 2 cases of Della Marca and colleagues[19] and Bejot and colleagues,[20] respectively, produce a total of 27 cases of sleep sex. Of these 27, 17 (63%) are reported with a personal history of non-REM parasomnia; mostly sleepwalking, sometimes combined with confusional arousal behavior, or sleep talking (however, sleep talking without association with another sleep disorder under the ICSD second edition 2005 is not classified as a parasomnia but as one of the isolated symptoms, apparently normal variants, and unresolved issues). Nineteen of the 27 combined cases (70%) were men, and 6 (all men) of the 27 (22%) had legal issues related to the sleep sex behavior.

In the Guilleminault and colleagues[5] series, 3 of the 11 cases were diagnosed after further investigations as having REM sleep behavior disorder as the sole other sleep disorder diagnosis, and there was 1 RBD case from Della Marca and colleagues.[19] Some investigators have discussed the problematic issue of RBD-associated sleep sex, given the documentation of hundreds of RBD cases without sexual acting-out, and the lack of such behavior in animal RBD models.[8] In the same Guilleminault and colleagues[5] series, 1 case was diagnosed as having stage 2 complex partial seizure disorder with EEG localization to

a mesiofrontal locus as the sole sleep disorder diagnosis associated with sleep sex. Schenck and colleagues[8] identified another 6 epilepsy-related instance of sleep sex.

The Shapiro and colleagues[3] case series contained 9 of 11 cases with ancillary features of non-REM parasomnia preceding or accompanying the sleep sex behavior. In 1 of these 9, sleeptalking was the only reported manifestation of a parasomnia-like behavior and, in this case, PSG support for a diagnosis of parasomnia was limited to intrusions of α activity into SWS and SWS arousals. Another of these 9 cases was a man who had been charged with sexual assault related to his digital vaginal penetration of an adjacent sleeping minor. Heavy alcohol consumption, and marijuana use, had occurred on the relevant night. Preceding parasomnia history in this instance was described by sleeptalking, and only 1 instance of sleepwalking.

In abstract form, Hurwitz and colleagues[17] presented 1 case of sleep sex behavior associated with sleep disordered breathing (SDB). Another case of sleep sex while snoring described by Rosenfeld and Elhajjar[2] suggests a possible association between sleep sex and SDB but, in that case, there was no PSG documentation of OSA, nor introduction of CPAP. In addition, Shapiro and colleagues[3] describe 1 case of sleep sex with PSG features of both non-REM parasomnia and OSA, with OSA likely playing a direct role in the sleep sex behavior; introduction and use of CPAP was associated with reported remission of the sleep sex behavior and subsequent withdrawal of CPAP was associated with its recurrence, with cessation of the behavior again on resumption of CPAP. Another case from the same series by Shapiro and colleagues[3] is reported as having upper airway resistance syndrome but without further detail. Della Marca and colleagues[19] also reported a case of OSA-related sleep sex behavior. Beyond these limited case reports of sleep sex linked to SDB, a study linking sleepwalking and concurrent SDB in young adults (some cases manifested only a subtle form of SDB, the upper airway resistance syndrome, with normal apnea-hypopnea index metric), with remission of the sleepwalking with effective treatment of the SDB,[30] may hypothetically have analogous pathophysiologic and treatment implications for non-REM parasomnia sleep sex behavior associated with the concurrent presence of SDB.

In a 2008 review in this journal, Plante and Winkelman[31] discussed the psychiatric considerations of parasomnias and referred to the potential role in the differential diagnosis of unusual parasomnia activity (including sleep sex and sleep-related violence) of the sleep-related dissociative disorders (SRDDs). ICSD second edition 2005 lists SRDD as the first category in the group Other Parasomnias. The dissociative disorders occur when there is "a disruption of the usually integrated functions of consciousness, memory, identity, or perception of the environment." Nocturnal episodes of dissociation may occur in about 25% of patients with dissociative disorders: these arise from well-established EEG wakefulness near sleep onset or after waking from established sleep, but, at least at initial presentation, may seem to be arising from sleep or to be sleep-related.[32] Daytime dissociative disorder and a history of physical and/or sexual abuse are a common, but not invariable, element. The Motet historical case referenced by Thoinot[13] relates an incident that occurred in 1880, and is likely to have represented an instance of a prolonged dissociative state with sexual elements (see Fenwick[26]). A more recent single case report (abstract) of elaborate sexual behavior attributable to SRDD supports the notion that the SRDDs may need consideration among the differential diagnoses of sleep sex.[33]

Because the strongest association of sleep sex is with the non-REM parasomnias, and some investigators posit that sleep sex (without association with another identifiable sleep disorder) is a variant of the non-REM parasomnias confusional arousals and sleepwalking, it is appropriate to consider the possible linkage between medication (and substance) use and sleep sex. Sleepwalking and other non-REM parasomnias have been linked in psychiatric populations to a range of and/or combinations of medications (eg, lithium carbonate, neuroleptics such as thioridazine, antidepressants such as paroxetine). In nonpsychiatric populations, the hypnotics triazolam and, particularly, the nonbenzodiazepam zolpidem have been reported to be associated with the occurrence of sleepwalking and variants thereof (eg, sleep-related eating disorder and sleep driving[34]). However, there are limited published data ascribing sleep sex behavior to medication use: zolpidem in 3 cases,[35,36] and the SSRI escitalopram in another.[37] In the 2003 series by Shapiro and colleagues,[3] 4 cases were described with a history, respectively, of multiple-substance abuse (in remission) and caffeine abuse, alcohol and marijuana use, past multiple-substance and alcohol abuse, and past alcohol abuse. However, the drug, alcohol, and substance associations cannot be taken to indicate any causal link to the sleep sex behavior of interest. Although alcohol and drug ingestion has been suggested as a precipitating factor for sexsomnia,[25] the evidence supporting this notion is scant; the role of alcohol as a primer or precipitant for sleepwalking and other non-REM parasomnias, whether associated with violence or not, is not supported by the published evidence.[38,39]

In addition, malingering needs consideration as a cause for apparent sleep sex behavior. This is discussed later.

Psychiatric comorbidity is a common reported feature of the case series discussed earlier. In the Guilleminault and colleagues[5] series depression (3), obsessive compulsive personality trait (2), and anxiety disorders (2) were present in 7 of the 11 cases but were not overtly linked by the investigators to the sleep sex behavior. In the Shapiro and colleagues[3] series, paraphilia (1), depression and posttraumatic stress disorder (1), schizophrenia (1), and developmental delay (1) were described associations in 4 subjects but it seems that data were lacking in 5 other subjects. Again, the investigators did not attribute these psychiatric comorbidities in a causative way directly to the sleep sex behaviors. Both of the 2 cases reported by Bejot and colleagues[20] had significant psychiatric comorbidity (obsessive compulsive personality trait; major depressive disorder and borderline personality trait).

DIAGNOSTIC APPROACH AND INVESTIGATIONS

As with all parasomnias and other abnormal sleep-related behaviors, and especially with putative non-REM parasomnias presenting with sleep sex behaviors, the key role of a full, accurate, and, where possible, corroborated history is paramount. A full medical, psychiatric, and social and family history should cover all details that may possibly affect the diagnostic process. Special attention should be given to consideration of the possible causal entities, and interviewers should remain open to the presentation of new causes. Physical examination should be comprehensive, with particular attention to signs of upper airway anatomic compromise. Formal psychiatric evaluation is mandated.

Specific investigations may be informed by historical or examination findings. The role of overnight video-polysomnography (PSG) is not to anticipate documentation of a sleep sex episode but to document, if present, the concurrence of other sleep disorders such as SDB or RBD. Although there have been many references in the literature to the characteristic (nonbehavioral) PSG features of sleepwalking and other non-REM parasomnias, the presence in an overnight PSG of abrupt arousals from SWS, hypersynchronous δ waves,[40] δ wave clusters, and increased or abnormal cyclic alternating pattern rate[41] are not pathognomonic features that, in post hoc application, should definitively sway an adjudication about a prior putative sleep-related event. An extended EEG montage PSG is indicated if sleep epilepsy is being considered, as are other epilepsy-specific investigations (eg, brain imaging, sleep-deprived EEG studies). Urine drug testing is appropriate. Extended electromyogram (EMG) montage should be considered when RBD is a diagnostic consideration. Particularly in difficult cases of diagnosis, referral to a laboratory and personnel skilled and experienced in assessing such cases should be considered.

In one of the case series described earlier, home studies played a part in the diagnostic and investigative process.[5] Home studies may include EEG and EMG monitoring or similar, audio recording, actimetry, and home video recording. Corroboration from a bed/sleep partner of events so recorded is important in these circumstances.

MANAGEMENT

Best management of individual cases of sleep sex is predicated on the most accurate causal diagnosis. Although a causal basis may have to be inferred by process of attempted exclusion of alternatives, in some instances a firm basis to the sleep sex behavior can be established. Treatment intervention then follows logically to address the underlying disorder that promotes the sleep sex behavior. Thus, if OSA is attributable, treatments such as CPAP or other effective OSA remedies can be applied. If RBD is the assumed basis of sleep sex, conventional treatment of RBD may involve administration of a benzodiazepine such as clonazepam, or an alternative RBD therapy like melatonin (although there is no published report of successful use of melatonin in a case of sleep sex). For dissociative disorders manifesting with sleep sex, the major therapeutic approach is via psychotherapeutic interventions.

In the most common situation of non-REM parasomnia sleep sex, the most effective therapy reported in the literature has been the benzodiazepine clonazepam. Its mode of action is not well understood when it is effectively used in the broader field of non-REM parasomnias, but it may act by state-stabilization mechanisms. Practical use of clonazepam in this context follows similar usage in non–sleep sex cases of non-REM parasomnia therapy, although there is a paucity of good evidence of efficacy[42]; other benzodiazepines may also be useful. In the limited number of published cases, other medications, such as SSRI antidepressants, are reported to have had some success (but there is a published case of SSRI-induced sleep sex[37]). The work of Guilleminault and colleagues[30] linking, in young adults, the non-REM parasomnia sleepwalking to often subtle degrees of SDB, and the described beneficial effects on the sleepwalking of effective treatment of the SDB, suggests that strenuous efforts should be directed to considering the possible presence of such SDB in patients who perform sleep sex.

PATHOPHYSIOLOGY

Knowledge of the underlying pathophysiology of sleep sex is largely conceptual. Logically, across the range of causal bases to sleep sex behavior, there may be a variety of driving pathophysiologic factors at play. In at least some of these, there may be interplay between well-described processes, for example the pathophysiology of the respiratory events and associated arousals of SDB in OSA, and the predisposed and perhaps primed brain of the individual with a preexisting history of tendency to non-REM parasomnia. In the sleep state, these diverse factors may align with the functional activation of specific neuroanatomic areas concerned with sex behavior. It is likely that the specifics of that functional neuroanatomic activation may also vary according to the type and degree of expression of different sleep sex behaviors, and to other factors including duration and affective elements.

This article does not review the underlying pathophysiologic aspects of arousals associated with respiratory events in OSA, or the mechanisms of epilepsy-related sleep sex behaviors. It is also beyond the scope of this article to explore further understanding of dissociative disorders. Because, numerically, sleep sex is mostly associated with non-REM parasomnia, it may help to reference what is known about the pathophysiology of non-REM parasomnia more commonly manifesting as sleepwalking or confusional arousal.

The understanding of the pathophysiology of non-REM parasomnia behavior generally is not comprehensively described, but there are some data to support generally accepted underlying concepts regarding non-REM parasomnia behavior. Genetic predisposition, and factors like sleep deprivation that prime the predisposed brain to be more susceptible to non-REM parasomnia behavior such as sleepwalking, allied to on-the-night acute precipitating factors such as touch or noise, promote the abrupt arousal from deep sleep that leads to the sleepwalking behavior.[38] Neuroimaging documentation of the brain's functional status at the time of such a parasomnia episode has been published in a single case by Bassetti and colleagues.[43] This study showed locoregional blood flow changes (using single-photon emission computed tomography [SPECT]) during the event consistent with metabolic quiescence of associative cortical areas and contemporaneous activation of limbic subcortical structures at/adjacent to the posterior cingulate gyrus. This study, and others not using direct functional imaging techniques (eg, sleepwalking events fortuitously captured on PSG or extended EEG recording), supports the concept of sleepwalking being a mixed state of partial sleep and partial wake.

Although the peripheral physiology of (at least male) wake human sexual behavior has been extensively studied (the sexual response cycle), and with ongoing exploration of neurochemical and other mediators of expression of sexual behavior,[44,45] the central neuroanatomic functional correlates of that behavior and other associated aspects of human sexual behavior have only recently been described with modern neuroimaging techniques. Ferretti and colleagues[46] described functional magnetic resonance imaging (fMRI) neuroanatomic localizations of interest: "activation maps highlighted a complex neural circuit involved in sexual arousal…only a few areas (anterior cingulate, insula, amygdala, hypothalamus, and secondary somatosensory cortices) were specifically correlated with penile erection…these areas showed distinct dynamic relationships with the time course of sexual response." No opportunity has arisen (and been published) so far to study functional neuroimaging aspects of sleep sex behavior. Such a study might indicate a complex association of inactive cortical areas, analogous to areas depicted in Bassetti and colleagues[43] SPECT study, aligned in time with activated sex-associated subcortical areas including the cingulated gyrus, amygdale, and hypothalamus.

In their review of the neurologic control of wake human sexual behavior, and taking into account data from lesion and stimulation studies, as well as from neuroimaging, Baird and colleagues[47] summarized 6 specific areas of interest in human sexual behavior: 3 were at the subcortical level, and 3 at the cortical level. At the cortical level is listed the frontal cortex associated with the motor control of sexual behavior, and the control of sexual response, which implies an array of activations and inactivations at the cortical and subcortical level for parasomnia behavior characterized by sleep sex. This array makes any conceptual construction of the pathophysiology of sleep sex in the non-REM parasomnia paradigm more complex: a possible combination of both cortical activation and cortical inactivation (of different cortical areas) combined with activation of other sex-associated subcortical levels, cascading to the peripheral manifestation of the sleep sex behavior.

Another component of the complex interplay in sleep between peripheral sexual behavioral phenomena and central neural activation of sex-associated cortical and subcortical areas that could play out in episodes of sleep sex may manifest in the putative roles of central pattern generators (CPG) and fixed action patterns. CPGs may be composed of aggregates of dedicated networks of neurons that, when activated, are responsible for the initiation, intensity, and persistence of complex motor behavior; such CPGs can be located in the brainstem in the vicinity of other complex neuronal collections that mediate state transitions between sleep and wake. Activation of appropriate CPGs may initiate the behavioral motor sequence that is recognized across species as the fixed action pattern. In a neuroethological approach to primitive sleep behaviors, Tassinari and colleagues[48] review this model in detail; it may provide a useful conceptual and experimental physiologic basis for parasomnias such as sleep sex (**Figs. 1** and **2**).

SOCIOCULTURAL ASPECTS OF SLEEP SEX

Published data on sleep sex have emanated from America, Europe, and Australasia. There has been

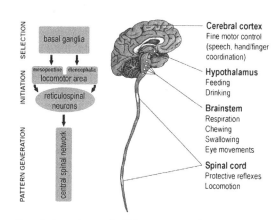

Fig. 1. Location of different CPG that coordinate different motor patterns/behaviors in vertebrates is shown on the right. The vertebrate control scheme for locomotion is shown on the left. The basal ganglia exert a tonic inhibitory influence on motor centers that is released when a motor pattern is selected. Locomotion is initiated by activity in reticulospinal neurons of the brainstem locomotor center, which produces a locomotor pattern modulated in the central spinal network. (*From* Tassinari CA, Rubboli G, Gardella E, et al. Central pattern generators for a common semiology in fronto-limbic seizures and in parasomnias. A neuroethologic approach. Neurol Sci 2005;26(Suppl 3):S225–32; with permission.)

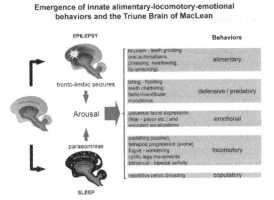

Emergence of innate alimentary-locomotory-emotional behaviors and the Triune Brain of MacLean

Fig. 2. Since 1952, the neurologist Paul MacLean proposed that the skull holds not 1 brain, but 3 (neo-mammalian, paleomammalian, and reptilian), each representing a distinct evolutionary stratum formed on the older layer before it, like an archaeological site. He calls it the triune brain (shown on the left). Both epilepsy and sleep can lead to a temporary loss of control of neomammalian cortex that facilitates, through a common platform (arousal), the emergences of motor events (shown in the middle) refer-able to stereotyped, inborn, fixed-action patterns (behaviors listed on the right). (*From* Tassinari CA, Rubboli G, Gardella E, et al. Central pattern generators for a common semiology in fronto-limbic seizures and in parasomnias. A neuroethologic approach. Neurol Sci 2005;26(Suppl 3):S225–32; with permission.)

no description of ethnic background in described cases. Although this limitation to a certain demo-graphic is likely more apparent than real, and related to levels of public and professional aware-ness, access to appropriate levels of professional care, religious and other cultural differences, studies to clarify any ethnic or other cultural pre-disposition would be of interest.

Despite its apparent infrequency, sleep sex gains considerable public attention, and that attention often spreads beyond national borders, when dramatic (often with a medicolegal context) cases are reported in the media. The idea of sleep sex has also gained currency in popular vehicles of mass culture such as television shows and feature movies. One possible consequence of this dissemination of the existence and idea of sleep sex may be more cases presenting within legal jurisdictions in countries where such media presentations are experienced by accused individ-uals and their legal counsels.

FORENSIC ASPECTS OF SLEEP SEX

A comprehensive review of the forensic aspects of sleep medicine and the particular treatment of sleep sex within that context is beyond the scope

of this article. A succinct and forward-looking overview of sleep forensics has been provided by Cramer Bornemann and Mahowald.[49] Some particular aspects of sleep sex in the forensic domain are presented here.

In a specific country/jurisdiction(s), when there are more cases presenting to the courts than have been published in local scientific journals, it might be reasonable to wonder sceptically about the apparently skewed distribution of such sleep sex cases. In addition, when sleep sex is pre-sented as a significant exculpating factor in acquittal decisions, it is not necessarily appro-priate in a scientific sense (without further supportive data) to ascribe that particular case to a definitive category of sleep sex behavior. Courts arrive at acquittal decisions for a range of reasons, many of which may not be related to the presented expert medical evidence. In some cases of puta-tive automatism caused by non-REM parasomnia sleep sex, critical evidence may be presented in the courts in a "she-said he-said" conflict of evidence without third-party corroboration, and it is then left to the jury/judge to ponder and pontifi-cate, and they may do so on other grounds than expert testimony, including the respective as-sessed credibility of the principal witness and accused. Similarly, in a scientific sense, conviction decisions in sleep sex court cases do not neces-sarily attest to a particular malingering cause.

Malingering has been defined as "the intentional production of false or grossly exaggerated phys-ical or psychological symptoms, motivated by external incentives...."[11] Malingering may be prevalent in offenders.[50,51] In medicolegal sleep sex cases, Ebrahim and Shapiro[52] recommend a forensic approach beyond that applied in clinical cases: emphasis should be given to careful exam-ination of the detail of the alleged offender's first account of the event (usually as recorded in police interviews), and heightened suspicion for malin-gering should be applied if the charged episode is the first described sleep sex/sleepwalking/para-somnia act known to have occurred for the indi-vidual, and when the alleged offender's recall varies between repeated evaluations. Prolonged periods of intense professional observation of the alleged offender in custody is a suggested, but possibly an impractical, extension to detailed indi-vidual assessment.

Principles of expert witness evidence giving in sleep sex cases are based on a rejection of the presentation of junk science to the court and a nonpartisan approach by the expert witness.[53,54] Professional bodies representing those likely to be engaged as sleep sex expert witnesses have recom-mended science-based ethical approaches.[55,56] In the area of sleep-related violence caused by possible automatism related to a non-REM parasomnia episode, from the perspective of the expert medical witness presenting evidence to a court, there are proposed guidelines[23,57,58] that encompass a multipoint appraisal of details of the individual and the violent act(s) (**Box 3**). Although this is of undoubted usefulness in the assessment of the accused by the medical expert, the relative weighting of specific positive, negative, or neutral criteria remains for the expert witness to decide, and the guideline approach has not been systematically tested.

A similar approach, but adapted for the sleep sex context, has been suggested by Trajanovic and Shapiro[29] and carries similar advantages and limitations. This guideline approach is specifically constructed for consideration of the non-REM parasomnia cause of sleep sex. Cramer Bornemann and Mahowald describe the dilemma that may challenge the expert medical witness in such cases.[49] Often enough, on the balance of evidence it is certainly possible that the complex behavior for which the accused is charged may well have occurred during a mixed state of wakefulness and sleep without full consciousness, but whether that actually is what occurred on the night in question can never be determined with certainty after the fact. Happily or otherwise for the expert witness, that determination in the legal domain is ultimately left to the court process.

As in forensic cases of sleep-related violence (sleep sex in the forensic context could be regarded as a particular subcategory of sleep-related violence), among all the other factors, the impact of alcohol (and other drugs, mostly illicit) may often need consideration. Alcohol intoxication behavior may superficially present some of the behavioral features of parasomnia behavior and, if occurring at night in appropriate circumstances, may be put forward by counsel as an automatism defense. The concept of alcohol or alcohol intoxication causing, de novo, the appearance of true parasomnia behavior has no evidence-based scientific foundation. The proposal that alcohol, or other illicit drugs (such as cannabis), promoting parasomnia behavior in a subject with a background of past parasomnia behavior such as sleepwalking also lacks any sound evidence base to date, as discussed earlier. Voluntary alcohol (or other drug) intoxication cannot be a complete defense in such criminal court proceedings. In this regard, the 2006 case described by Ebrahim[59] is troubling because of the prominent role of alcohol in the events of the night in question and on prior alleged sleepwalking events attributed to the defendant, as is the use of "a popular method" of alcohol challenge before the overnight sleep study. There has been no scientific validation of the so-called alcohol challenge sleep study in the context of supposed effects of alcohol on the sleep of sleepwalkers[60,61] or subjects engaging in sleep sex behavior.

Variations in the legal processes across international jurisdictions, interpretations of what constitutes automatism, the legal concepts of actus reus and mens rea, approaches defining consciousness, and neuroethological ideas like fixed action patterns and central pattern generators are established and evolving concepts that are more fully addressed in appropriate sources covering contemporary neuroscience and forensic sleep medicine.[49,52]

Box 3
Guidelines for assessing episodes of sleep sex behavior in the forensic context and applicable to non-REM parasomnia sleep sex

- Good reasons to consider preexisting bona fide sleep disorder (such reasons might include previous adequate medical documentation of sleep disorder) and history of similar sleep sex episodes with benign or morbid outcome having been reasonably documented to have occurred before the alleged event

- Brief duration of action (<20–30 minutes)

- Relevant behavior is abrupt, immediate, impulsive, senseless, without apparent premotivation

- Inappropriate to the total situation, out of waking character for the individual, lacking evidence of premeditation

- Victim is often someone who happened to be present

- With return to full consciousness, and if made aware of the events, there is perplexity/horror and no attempt to escape or conceal the behavior

- If available, other witness corroboration indicates lack of awareness on the part of the individual during the sleep sex act(s)

- Amnesia pertains to the event, although this may be partial

- Typically occurs within 1–2 hours of sleep onset (if known), is associated with physical contact in bed with a bed partner, and is promoted or precipitated by acceptable factors (eg, prior sleep deprivation)

Modified from Cramer Bornemann MA, Mahowald MW. Sleep forensics. In: Principles and practice of sleep medicine. 5th edition. Philadelphia: Elsevier Saunders; 2011. p. 725–33. Chapter 63.

SUMMARY

Sleep sex is an uncommon problem encountered in most sleep medicine and other clinical practices. A common pathway of sexual behavior in sleep may result from diverse pathophysiologic processes, and the most commonly attributable associated sleep disorders are the non-REM parasomnia entities, confusional arousal, and sleepwalking. Research of sleep sex is in its infancy: further efforts to document the true prevalence of this disorder in various communities, to delineate the functional neuroanatomic areas of interest and their interconnectedness, and to best define the various treatment options, will enhance the scientific basis of this arcane field of sleep medicine.

There are often challenges to establishing whether a sexual act has occurred in/from sleep, or merely has occurred in a night-time sleep-suggested setting. In forensic sleep medicine, the contribution of sleep medicine science should follow established principles of expert witness evidence giving, be rigorously science based, and take heed of evolving knowledge in neuroscience and related fields. There is always a need to admit limitation to true knowledge of the nature of such events when addressed in a post hoc manner.

REFERENCES

1. Alves R, Aloe F, Tavares S, et al. Sexual behavior in sleep, sleepwalking and possible REM behavior disorder: a case report. Sleep Res Online 1999;2(3):71–2.

2. Rosenfeld DS, Elhajjar AJ. Sleepsex: a variant of sleepwalking. Arch Sex Behav 1998;27(3):269–78.

3. Shapiro CM, Trajanovic NN, Fedoroff JP. Sexsomnia–a new parasomnia? Can J Psychiatry 2003; 48(5):311–7.

4. Trajanovic NN, Mangan M, Shapiro CM. Sexual behaviour in sleep: an internet survey. Soc Psychiatry Psychiatr Epidemiol 2007;42(12):1024–31.

5. Guilleminault C, Moscovitch A, Yuen K, et al. Atypical sexual behavior during sleep. Psychosom Med 2002;64(2):328–36.

6. Schmidt MH. Neural mechanisms of sleep related penile erections. In: Kryger MH, Roth T, Dement WC, editors. Principles and practice of sleep medicine. 4th edition. Philadelphia: Elsevier Saunders; 2005.

7. Karsenty G, Werth E, Knapp PA, et al. Sleep-related painful erections. Nat Clin Pract Urol 2005;2(5): 256–60 [quiz: 261].

8. Schenck CH, Arnulf I, Mahowald MW. Sleep and sex: what can go wrong? A review of the literature on sleep related disorders and abnormal sexual behaviors and experiences. Sleep 2007;30(6): 683–702.

9. Szucs A, Janszky J, Hollo A, et al. Misleading hallucinations in unrecognized narcolepsy. Acta Psychiatr Scand 2003;108(4):314–6 [discussion: 316–7].

10. American Academy of Sleep Medicine. International classification of sleep disorders: diagnostic and coding manual. 2nd edition. Westchester (IL): American Academy of Sleep Medicine; 2005.

11. American Psychiatric Association. Diagnostic and statistical manual of mental disorders. text revision (DSM-IV-TR). 4th edition. Arlington (VA): American Psychiatric Association; 2000.

12. World Health Organization. International classification of disease, 10th revision. Albany (NY): World Health Organization; 2007.

13. Thoinot L. Medicolegal aspects of moral offenders. Philadelphia: David and Company; 1911.

14. Langeluddeke A. Delicts in sleeping states. Nervenarzt 1955;26(1):28–30 [in German].

15. Hartman E. Two case reports: night terrors with sleepwalking - a potentially lethal disorder. J Nerv Ment Dis 1983;171(8):503–5.

16. Wong KE. Masturbation during sleep–a somnambulistic variant? Singapore Med J 1986;27(6):542–3.

17. Hurwitz TD, Mahowald MH, Schluter JL. Sleep-related sexual abuse of children. Sleep Res 1989; 18:246.

18. Buchanan A. Sleepwalking and indecent exposure. Med Sci Law 1991;31(1):38–40.

19. Della Marca G, Dittoni S, Frusciante R, et al. Abnormal sexual behavior during sleep. J Sex Med 2009;6(12):3490–5.

20. Bejot Y, Juenet N, Garrouty R, et al. Sexsomnia: an uncommon variety of parasomnia. Clin Neurol Neurosurg 2010;112(1):72–5.

21. Kennedy GA, Elzo F. Case studies of familial sexsomnia. Sleep Biol Rhythm 2010;8:A73–4.

22. Mangan MA, Reips UD. Sleep, sex, and the Web: surveying the difficult-to-reach clinical population suffering from sexsomnia. Behav Res Methods 2007;39(2):233–6.

23. Ohayon MM, Caulet M, Priest RG. Violent behavior during sleep. J Clin Psychiatry 1997;58(8):369–76 [quiz: 377].

24. Chung SA, Yegneswaran B, Natarajan A, et al. Frequency of sexsomnia in sleep clinic patients. Sleep 2010;33(abstract supplement):A226.

25. Andersen ML, Poyares D, Alves RS, et al. Sexsomnia: abnormal sexual behavior during sleep. Brain Res Rev 2007;56(2):271–82.

26. Fenwick P. Sleep and sexual offending. Med Sci Law 1996;36(2):122–34.

27. Zadra A, Pilon M, Montplaisir J. Polysomnographic diagnosis of sleepwalking: effects of sleep deprivation. Ann Neurol 2008;63(4):513–9.

28. Pilon M, Montplaisir J, Zadra A. Precipitating factors of somnambulism: impact of sleep deprivation and forced arousals. Neurology 2008;70(24):2284–90.

29. Trajanovic NN, Shapiro CM. Sexsomnias. Cambridge (United Kingdom): Cambridge University Press; 2010.

30. Guilleminault C, Kirisoglu C, Bao G, et al. Adult chronic sleepwalking and its treatment based on polysomnography. Brain 2005;128(Pt 5):1062–9.

31. Plante DT, Winkelman JW. Parasomnias: psychiatric considerations. Sleep Med Clin 2008;3(2):217–29.

32. Schenck CH, Milner DM, Hurwitz TD, et al. Dissociative disorders presenting as somnambulism: polysomnographic, video and clinical documentation (8 cases). Dissociation 1989;11(4):194–204.

33. Buchanan PR. Sleep sex behaviour: an underreported parasomnia? Int Med J 2005;35(Suppl): A27.

34. Pressman MR. Sleep driving: sleepwalking variant or misuse of z-drugs? Sleep Med Rev 2011;15(5): 285–92.

35. Schenck CH, Connoy DA, Castellanos M, et al. Zolpidem-induced amnestic sleep-related eating disorder (SRED) in 19 patients. Sleep 2005; 28(Abstract Supplement):A259.

36. Schenck CH. Paradox lost: midnight in the battleground of sleep and dreams. Minneapolis (MN): Extreme-Nights, LLC; 2005.

37. Krol DG. Sexsomnia during treatment with a selective serotonin reuptake inhibitor. Tijdschr Psychiatr 2008; 50(11):735–9 [in Dutch].

38. Pressman MR. Factors that predispose, prime and precipitate NREM parasomnias in adults: clinical and forensic implications. Sleep Med Rev 2007; 11(1):5–30 [discussion: 31–3].

39. Pressman MR, Mahowald MW, Schenck CH, et al. Alcohol-induced sleepwalking or confusional arousal as a defense to criminal behavior: a review of scientific evidence, methods and forensic considerations. J Sleep Res 2007;16(2):198–212.

40. Pressman MR. Hypersynchronous delta sleep EEG activity and sudden arousals from slow-wave sleep in adults without a history of parasomnias: clinical and forensic implications. Sleep 2004;27(4): 706–10.

41. Guilleminault C, Kirisoglu C, da Rosa AC, et al. Sleepwalking, a disorder of NREM sleep instability. Sleep Med 2006;7(2):163–70.

42. Harris M, Grunstein RR. Treatments for somnambulism in adults: assessing the evidence. Sleep Med Rev 2009;13(4):295–7.

43. Bassetti C, Vella S, Donati F, et al. SPECT during sleepwalking. Lancet 2000;356(9228):484–5.

44. Andersson KE. Erectile physiological and pathophysiological pathways involved in erectile dysfunction. J Urol 2003;170(2 Pt 2):S6–13 [discussion: S13–4].

45. de Groat WC. Autonomic nervous system: urogenital control. Academic Press, Elsevier; 2009.

46. Ferretti A, Caulo M, Del Gratta C, et al. Dynamics of male sexual arousal: distinct components of brain activation revealed by fMRI. Neuroimage 2005; 26(4):1086–96.

47. Baird AD, Wilson SJ, Bladin PF, et al. Neurological control of human sexual behaviour: insights from lesion studies. J Neurol Neurosurg Psychiatry 2007;78(10):1042–9.

48. Tassinari CA, Rubboli G, Gardella E, et al. Central pattern generators for a common semiology in fronto-limbic seizures and in parasomnias. A neuroethologic approach. Neurol Sci 2005;26(Suppl 3): s225–32.

49. Cramer Bornemann MA, Mahowald MW. Sleep forensics. In: Kryger MH, Roth T, Dement WC, editors. Principles and practice of sleep medicine. 5th edition. Philadelphia: Elsevier Saunders; 2011. p. 725–33. Chapter 63.

50. Rogers R, Sewell KW, Morey LC, et al. Detection of feigned mental disorders on the personality assessment inventory: a discriminant analysis. J Pers Assess 1996;67(3):629–40.

51. Pollock PH, Quigley B, Worley KO, et al. Feigned mental disorder in prisoners referred to forensic mental health services. J Psychiatr Ment Health Nurs 1997;4(1):9–15.

52. Ebrahim IO, Shapiro CM. Medico-legal consequences of parasomnias. Cambridge (United Kingdom): Cambridge University Press; 2010.

53. Mahowald MW, Schenck CH, Cramer-Bornemann M. Finally–sleep science for the courtroom. Sleep Med Rev 2007;11(1):1–3.

54. Buchanan PR, King PJ, Grunstein RR. Commentary on "Factors that predispose, prime and precipitate NREM parasomnias in adults: clinical and forensic implications". Sleep Med Rev 2007;11(1):31–3.

55. Cramer Bornemann MA. Role of the expert witness in sleep-related violence trials. American Medical Association Journal of Ethics: Virtual Mentor 2008; 10(9):571–7.

56. American Academy of Neurology. Qualifications and guidelines for the physician expert witness. Available at: http://www.aan.com/go/about/position/Physician Expert Witness. Accessed April 2, 2011.

57. Bonkalo A. Impulsive acts and confusional states during incomplete arousal from sleep: criminological and forensic implications. Psychiatr Q 1974;48(3): 400–9.

58. Mahowald MW, Bundlie SR, Hurwitz TD, et al. Sleep violence–forensic science implications: polygraphic and video documentation. J Forensic Sci 1990; 35(2):413–32.

59. Ebrahim IO. Somnambulistic sexual behaviour (sexsomnia). J Clin Forensic Med 2006;13(4):219–24.

60. Ebrahim IO, Fenwick P. Sleep-related automatism and the law. Med Sci Law 2008;48(2):124–36.

61. Pressman MR, Mahowald MH, Schenck CH, et al. Letters to the editor, including response from the authors. Med Sci Law 2009;49(2):139–49.

Sleep Eating

Michael J. Howell, MD[a,b],*

KEYWORDS

- Sleep-related eating disorder • Restless legs syndrome
- Parasomnia • Sleepwalking

This article first addresses the physiology that maintains the normal overnight fast. The clinical characteristics of sleep-related eating disorder (SRED) are then described, with a focus on the association with restless legs syndrome as well as sedative-hypnotic medications as a contributor to amnestic eating. The relationships between nocturnal eating and obesity are considered. Although treatment trials are still in their infancy, the initial reports are reviewed. Please see **Table 1** for definitions used in this article.

NORMAL METABOLIC PHYSIOLOGY DURING SLEEP

Under normal conditions the nocturnal period in humans is typically characterized by a prolonged period of fasting for approximately half of every 24-hour day. However, energy homeostasis is maintained through alterations in glucose regulation and appetite modulation, in contrast to fasting during sedentary wakefulness, which demonstrates progressive hypoglycemia and hunger over 12 hours.[1]

During constant glucose infusion (which eliminates confounding meal timing factors), serum glucose levels are high during both nighttime sleep and daytime naps.[1] Several changes in systemic and cerebral glucose use and tolerance help maintain these stable energy stores during sleep. First, diminished motor activity that characterizes sleep contributes to decreased peripheral metabolism. Second, brain metabolism of glucose is reduced during sleep, particularly during non–rapid-eye-movement (NREM) sleep, for which positron emission tomography (PET) studies have demonstrated a 40% reduction

central nervous system (CNS) metabolism.[2,3] Third, insulin is rapidly disposed of during sleep, resulting in more available glucose.[4] Fourth, growth hormone (GH) is secreted with sleep onset, stimulating hepatic gluconeogenesis and inhibiting glucose uptake.[5] Sleep deprivation suppresses GH secretion until sleep is initiated, regardless of the circadian period.[5] Sleep-onset GH secretion is also associated with increasing density of slow-wave sleep.[6] This relationship allows for anabolic processes to occur during periods of musculoskeletal and cerebral quiescence. Finally, cortisol secretion near the end of the sleep period stimulates gluconeogenesis, promotes lipolysis, and mobilizes amino acids and ketones.[5]

Sleep changes in hormone secretion promote satiety and suppresses appetite. In particular, leptin, a peptide hormone secreted by adipocytes, inhibits hunger centers in the hypothalamus. Leptin peaks soon after sleep onset, helping to suppress feeding behavior.[7] Conversely the hormone ghrelin, which is a hunger signal, has increased levels during sleep in humans.[8] Presumably, therefore, during sleep there is a balance between increased ghrelin and increased leptin activity that does not promote eating.

Despite a prolonged fast, energy homeostasis is thus maintained during sleep through alterations in glucose metabolism and appetite regulation, as listed in **Table 2**.

DEFINITION OF SLEEP-RELATED EATING DISORDER

SRED was originally described in 1991, and is defined as a parasomnia (abnormal behavior at

The author has nothing to disclose.
a Department of Neurology, University of Minnesota, 717 Delaware Street SE, Room 510, Minneapolis, MN 55455, USA
b Parasomnia Program, University of Minnesota Medical Center, Minneapolis, MN, USA
* Department of Neurology, University of Minnesota, 717 Delaware Street SE, Room 510, Minneapolis, MN 55455.
E-mail address: howel020@umn.edu

Sleep Med Clin 6 (2011) 429–439
doi:10.1016/j.jsmc.2011.07.002

Table 1
Definitions used in this article

Night eating	Eating after the evening meal and before final awakening
Evening hyperphagia	Excessive eating after the evening meal and before falling asleep
Nocturnal eating	Eating that occurs after an arousal from sleep before final awakening

night) with recurrent episodes of eating after an arousal from nighttime sleep with adverse consequences. The episodes are described as occurring in an involuntary, compulsive, or "out of control" manner. Patients often cannot be easily awakened, especially in the setting of sedative-hypnotic medications, and in this regard SRED resembles somnambulism.[9–11] SRED is not to be confused with the night eating syndrome (NES), described in 1955 by Stunkard and colleagues,[12] a circadian delay in meal timing resulting in evening hyperphagia, nocturnal eating, and morning anorexia. SRED shares many similarities with NES; however, it is distinguished by the presence of nocturnal eating alone without evening hyperphagia. For an excellent review of NES see Ref.[13]

EPIDEMIOLOGY

Epidemiologic studies suggest that nocturnal eating (both dysfunctional and nondysfunctional) and SRED (dysfunctional nocturnal eating alone) are common phenomena, particularly among patients with other sleep disorders. The most striking relationship is restless legs syndrome (RLS) and SRED. According to a survey of 53 RLS patients who presented to a sleep disorder center, 66% have frequent nocturnal eating and 45% have SRED.[14] These findings are similar to those of a survey of 100 RLS patients who demonstrated

a 33% prevalence of SRED.[15] These and other reports suggest a fundamental relationship between RLS and nocturnal eating (see the section "The Relationship Between SRED and RLS"). SRED is also frequently associated with other parasomnias. Three series have reported comorbid sleepwalking in 48% to 65% of patients with SRED.[9,10,16] Sleepwalking without eating may precede SRED and then, once nocturnal eating develops, it often becomes the predominant sleepwalking behavior.[9] The majority (60%–83%) of reported cases is female.[9,10,17] Amnestic SRED is typically associated with psychotropic medications, in particular sedative hypnotics (see the section "SRED and Benzodiazepine Receptor Agonists").

SRED is associated with psychiatric comorbidities. In the original 1991 case series 47% of SRED patients (9/19) had an Axis 1 disorder, and many had daytime anxiety about potentially choking or starting fires while asleep.[9] A more recent report noted that 40% (14/35) of patients with nocturnal eating met criteria for depressed mood,[17] while a separate study noted that patients with SRED endorsed more symptoms of depression and dissociation than those without SRED.[18] SRED has also been noted among eating disorder groups. A self-administered questionnaire determined prevalence rates of 16.7% in an inpatient eating disorder group, 8.7% in an outpatient eating disorder group, and 4.6% in an unselected group of college students.[18] This latter finding is similar to a survey of 1235 general psychiatry patients, which noted a 4% lifetime prevalence of SRED and a 2.4% 1-year prevalence.[19]

SRED is associated with weight gain and obesity; however, a causal relationship has not yet been established. In the original 1991 case series nearly half of all patients fulfilled established criteria for being overweight,[9] and in a follow-up report 44% of patients claimed that greater than 20% of their excess weight was related to nocturnal eating.[20]

CLINICAL CHARACTERISTICS

SRED is a relentless, chronic condition. In the original description of SRED, more than half (58%)

Table 2
Energy homeostasis during sleep

Decreased Glucose Use	Impaired Glucose Tolerance	Appetite Suppression
Decreased motor activity	Growth hormone secretion at sleep onset	Increased leptin (satiety hormone)
Decreased cerebral glucose activity (NREM sleep)	Insulin disposal increased Cortisol secretion during second half of sleep period	

described nocturnal eating at least once a night.[9] In another study the majority of patients described a long history of involuntary nocturnal eating (mean duration 16 years) and nearly all reported eating on a nightly basis.[10] A substantial proportion of SRED patients (23%) describe eating more than 5 times a night.[17]

SRED is characterized by consumption of high caloric foods, sometimes-dangerous food preparation, and the occasional ingestion of nonfood substances. The most commonly consumed foods are high in carbohydrates and fats. Of interest, hunger is notably absent with patients often describing a compulsion to eat so that sleep may be reinitiated.[10,17] Unconscious food preparation has resulted in injuries such as drinking excessively hot liquids, choking, and lacerations. Furthermore, inedible and toxic substances have been consumed, for example, egg shells, coffee grounds, sunflower shells, buttered cigarettes, glue, and cleaning solutions. Finally, patients have ingested foods to which they are allergic.[10,20,21]

Various medical consequences can occur from repeated nocturnal eating. Weight gain is commonly reported, and SRED may precipitate, or aggravate, diabetes mellitus, hyperlipidemia, hypercholesterolemia, hypertension, and obstructive sleep apnea.[10,20,21] Patients with SRED are at risk for dental caries, as dental hygiene practices rarely follow the feeding episodes.[20] Furthermore, many patients will fall asleep with an oral food bolus, which combined with the circadian decline in salivary flow leads to dental caries. Finally, failure to exhibit control over nocturnal eating can lead to secondary depressive disorders.[10]

Polysomnography (PSG) has been used to characterize SRED, with commonly consumed nocturnal food available at bedside to facilitate eating behavior. If a patient eats during the PSG study, the concomitant sleep-wake state is then identified and the technologist can assess the level of awareness at the time, and subsequently the patient's recall of the event in the morning. Similar to sleepwalking, the nocturnal events most commonly arise from NREM sleep. A recent study documented that 44 of 45 feeding episodes in 26 patients arose from NREM sleep. Elevated periodic limb movements and rhythmic masticatory muscle activity (RMMA) associated with arousal from NREM sleep have been reported in the majority of SRED cases studied with PSG.[17,20]

Early reports suggest that SRED may have a genetic predisposition. In one case a 31-year-old woman with SRED reported that her dizygotic twin sister and father were also affected.[22] Another study described that 26% (6/23) of SRED patients claimed to have a first-degree relative with nocturnal eating behavior.[10] By contrast, only 6% (2/36) of subjects described similar behaviors in family members in a separate report.[17] Additional research clearly is needed to determine whether nocturnal eating is an inherited trait.

SRED and Amnesia

The presence of impaired consciousness in the definition of SRED has evolved since its original description. Historically complete or at least partial unconsciousness was a defining feature of SRED. In the original series of SRED cases, 84% (32/38) of patients claimed at least partial impairment in awareness.[9] In another case series, 91% (21/23) of patients had incomplete consciousness and/or amnesia for the behavior.[10] Conversely, a subsequent study demonstrated full awareness during nocturnal eating episodes in all 26 patients after episodes of nocturnal eating in a sleep laboratory. However, the investigators did not report whether the subjects typically had full awareness during nocturnal eating at home.[17] This distinction is important, as the level of consciousness may be different in a sleep laboratory in comparison with a more familiar (ie, home) sleeping environment. Also, in SRED, awareness will vary night to night and sometimes between episodes of the same night.[23] Reduced awareness and subsequent amnesia is not a required diagnostic criterion for SRED in the International Classification of Sleep Disorders (2nd Edition),[11] even though most SRED patients do not claim full consciousness while engaged in nocturnal eating, especially in the setting of hypnotic medications.

The spectrum of amnesia noted in SRED reports may be explained by comorbid sleepwalking and by the use of sedating medication (see the section "SRED and Benzodiazepine Receptor Agonists").[17] The first case reports of nocturnal eating with amnesia were associated with comorbid sleepwalking disorders or with sedative psychotropic medications.[20,24,25] Moreover, the majority of patients in the original series was taking hypnotic medication or had a previous history of sleepwalking.[9] In a community survey of 92 subjects who admitted to nocturnal eating, only 18% reported they were at least partially unaware of the nocturnal eating. None of the participants who were fully aware of the events had a history of sleepwalking. By contrast, if subjects did have a sleepwalking history they were far more likely (73%) to be at least partially unaware of the behavior.[26] Finally, all 26 patients who demonstrated full consciousness during nocturnal eating episodes in a sleep laboratory were drug free, and only one had a history of sleepwalking.[17]

SRED and Benzodiazepine Receptor Agonists

Before the original SRED series in 1991, early case reports of amnestic nocturnal eating were associated with sedating psychotropic medications. These cases were often characterized by prolonged and dramatic sleepwalking with eating events.[27] More recently, SRED has been implicated with use of the benzodiazepine receptor agonists (BRA), in particular zolopidem.[28,29] In fact, the first case of amnestic nocturnal eating in 1981 was associated with a combination of chlorpromazine, amitriptyline, and methyprylon.[24] Subsequently SRED has been reported with triazolam, lithium, olanzapine, risperidone, zopiclone, and zaleplon.[16,20,30–32]

The majority of drug-induced SRED cases is related to zolpidem, a benzodiazepine receptor agonist. The first reported case of amnestic nocturnal eating related to zolpidem use was described in a member of the armed services in 1999.[33] A series comprising zolpidem-associated SRED followed in 2002. Five middle-aged patients were described, 2 of whom already had intermittent episodes of conscious nocturnal eating prior to starting zolpidem. All 5 patients were on various neuropsychiatric agents, and interestingly all had a history of RLS. Soon after initiating zolpidem, each patient described amnestic nocturnal eating that stopped with discontinuation.[28]

Further reports have strengthened the association between zolpidem and SRED. In a series of 1235 patients in an outpatient psychiatry clinic, the combination of zolpidem and antidepressants posed the greatest risk for SRED. In another report of 29 sleepwalkers in whom a high usage of BRA for sleep was noted (86%), 65.5% of patients described sleep-related eating behavior.[16] More recently, 8 patients reported that nocturnal eating began on average 40 days after starting zolpidem.[34] The vast majority of reports note improvement if not outright resolution of nocturnal eating behavior after the agents are discontinued.[28,33–37]

Extended-release formulations of zolpidem have also been implicated in SRED.[38,39] Of interest is one report that noted resolution in 2 patients once they were switched from extended-release to immediate-release zolpidem, demonstrating a striking interindividual variability.[39]

Uncontrollable nocturnal eating is often reported after patients ingest greater than the maximum recommended dose of zolpidem (10 mg).[29,40] Often this occurs when, in a desperate attempt to initiate sleep, patients escalate their dose without a new prescription.[29] Recently a cross-sectional pilot study of 125 psychiatric patients on hypnosedatives evaluated the risk factors for complex sleep behaviors such as amnestic sleep eating. Multiple regression analysis showed that a higher dose of zolpidem was the only significant predictor of complex sleep behaviors. Further, none of the subjects who demonstrated complex sleep behaviors took a dose of less than 10 mg.[41]

The spectrum of feeding behavior is diverse in SRED. A typical case report described a 51-year-old woman with RLS who noted empty food packages the mornings after she started taking zolpidem. She later discerned that she had been eating sandwiches on several occasions.[35] A more alarming example included prolonged amnestic behavior in a 45-year-old man. After 10 days of treatment, he was missing on two occasions after going to bed. Subsequently it was discovered that after driving his car over 2 km he had climbed into his place of business through the shutter to eat chocolate and other carbohydrate-rich snacks.[36]

BRAs enhance γ-aminobutyric acid (GABA) activity at central $GABA_A$ receptors, resulting in hypnotic phenomena such as sleep and amnesia. It has been suggested that the complex behavior noted with some BRAs is in part related to increasing binding affinity, and that zolpidem has the highest binding affinity among the BRA.[27,42]

Investigators have used functional neuroimaging to explore the neuropharmacologic mechanisms of drug-induced SRED. A case of zolpidem-induced SRED was studied with ^{18}F-fluorodeoxyglucose (FDG) PET during sleep while on and off zolpidem, but did not demonstrate significant differences in brain metabolism.[43] Of note, these findings are consistent with a larger FDG PET study that did not demonstrate metabolic differences during sleep in 12 normal volunteers studied while on and off zolpidem.[44]

As hypnotic agents suppress memory and executive function, it may be that zolpidem by itself does not activate SRED but instead disinhibits the behavior in a patient population at risk for nocturnal feeding. Patients with RLS demonstrate a greater tendency toward both dysfunctional and nondysfunctional nocturnal eating.[14,15] It is important that a substantial number of cases of BRA-associated amnestic nocturnal eating is seen in the setting of patients with RLS (see next section).[14,15,28,39,45]

The Relationship Between SRED and RLS

A critical review of both the SRED and RLS literature would suggest that there is an intimate relationship between these conditions. This conclusion is based on similarities in epidemiology, polysomnographic phenomena, clinical course, and treatment response. The evidence is especially compelling in cases of medication-induced SRED whereby the mistreatment of RLS as psychophysiological insomnia (PI) is plausible and, based on recent investigations, amnestic eating the expected result. Here the data supporting such a link are presented, with a summary conclusion at the end of the section.

RLS is common disorder affecting approximately 8% to 10% of the population, and is thus a common cause of sleep initiation and maintenance failure.[11,46,47] Furthermore, although RLS is distinct from PI, it is commonly confused with it. Thus it may be expected that many patients with RLS will be mistakenly treated with agents designed to treat PI.

Like SRED, RLS has a higher prevalence in women.[11,46] Unlike idiopathic sleepwalking, which demonstrates an equal gender distribution, medication-induced SRED is more common in women.[29,48]

Similar to RLS,[49] several features of SRED suggest an underlying dopamine dysfunction. First, dopamine mediates impulsive behaviors such as motor restlessness, smoking, and binge eating.[49,50] Second, a PSG study of 35 SRED patients demonstrated that 77% had PSG confirmation of wakeful RLS and periodic limb movement during sleep.[17] Third, RMMA, bruxism, and dopaminergic phenomena,[17,51] all associated with RLS,[52] are commonly seen in SRED.[17,20] In the original and follow-up SRED case series, prominent repetitive chewing movements were described during NREM sleep and after arousals.[9,20] In a recent study, RMMA was found in 29 of 35 patients diagnosed with SRED during their PSG evaluations.[17]

Two investigations demonstrated a high prevalence of both SRED and nondysfunctional nocturnal eating in patients with RLS. A community survey of 100 RLS patients revealed a high prevalence of SRED in RLS (33%) compared with normal population controls (1%).[15] The investigators pondered whether the compulsive nocturnal eating was related to underlying RLS brain pathology or whether nocturnal eating was merely "killing time" as previously suggested.[53] Another report of 80 patients with either RLS or PI who presented to a sleep disorders center noted that 66% of RLS patients described nocturnal eating and 45% had SRED. Conversely, only 7% of PI patients met criteria for SRED (no PI patients described nocturnal eating alone). This study suggests that nocturnal eating in RLS is not merely "killing time," as PI patients were more likely to have prolonged (>5 minutes) nightly awakenings (85%) compared with patients with RLS (30%), yet were much less likely to eat.[14]

Resembling the subclinical manifestation of SRED, that is, nondysfunctional nocturnal eating, RLS has mild forms that do not interfere with sleep onset.[54] Also, RLS is a difficult condition to diagnose, as current symptomatic criteria fail to identify many cases and atypical variants frequently go unrecognized during routine clinical evaluation.[55] Thus it may be expected that many cases of unrecognized RLS, or subclinical variations, exist in the SRED clinical population.

A fascinating case helps illustrate the intimate relationship between SRED and RLS. A 74-year-old woman presented 20 years ago with history of uncontrollable RLS and nocturnal eating. Both the nocturnal eating and RLS were well controlled with alpazolam, acetaminophen/codeine, and carbidopa/levodopa. Subsequently, ropinerol was added to fully control RLS. Then with the onset of a right lower extremity zoster eruption the patient had a relapse, with bilateral RLS as well as SRED. Compellingly, the patient's RLS and SRED resolved in parallel with the resolution of the skin lesions. Medications were not adjusted in the period immediately before, during, or after the zoster event.[56] Although the underlying mechanism in this case is unknown, iron-related proteins (iron is a catalyst in dopamine metabolism) are noted to change in the setting of herpetic infections.[57]

Intriguingly, the nocturnal feeding behavior of SRED closely resembles the motor activity of RLS. RLS is characterized by an underlying feeling (often poorly described) of discomfort in the lower extremities that compels the patient to move. Movement relieves the symptoms, although only temporarily, and sleep is unable to be reinitiated until this urge is addressed.[58] In SRED, patients state that after an awakening from sleep they have a compulsion to eat (often without hunger) that interferes with sleep maintenance. Subsequently, once food is ingested the feeling abates and sleep may be reinitiated.[11,15,20,59]

Compulsive nocturnal eating is not unexpected, as RLS patients often describe other nonmotor comorbidities such as mood and anxiety disorders and daytime smoking,[60–62] as well as other nocturnal compulsions that interfere with sleep, such as smoking.[59] It has even been suggested that the name itself be changed from RLS to Ekbom syndrome to recognize the various nonmotor manifestations of this condition.[63] Recently 6 cases of nocturnal eating and nocturnal smoking were reported. Five of the 6 cases either presented with or were noted to have RLS. Patients claimed that they would wake up and be unable to return to sleep without eating and/or smoking. In a follow-up study that investigated the prevalence of nocturnal smoking, RLS patients demonstrated an increase prevalence of nocturnal smoking (12%) compared with matched controls (2%). Of interest, among RLS patients with nocturnal smoking SRED was common (83%) and both phenomena often began simultaneously.[59] Moreover, patients with nonmotor phenomena of RLS have more severe motor restlessness as measured by the International RLS Rating Scale.[59]

It has been suggested that nocturnal eating and other nonmotor manifestations of RLS may be caused by dopaminergic agents, as these agents are known to trigger daytime impulsive behaviors such as gambling.[64–68] However, dopamine agents suppress feeding behavior in animal models,[69] and recent reports suggest that dopaminergic agents are not the cause of the nocturnal eating. In a survey of 33 patients with SRED and RLS, 10 patients reported that nocturnal eating emerged before or concomitant with RLS, and none reported that SRED emerged after the start of dopaminergic therapy. Also, RLS patients with SRED were not significantly more likely to use dopaminergic drugs than were RLS patients without SRED. In fact, subjects whose nocturnal eating symptoms were under control were more likely to be on these agents than subjects who continued to have nocturnal eating episodes.[15] Further, a double-blind treatment trial of pramipexole for SRED demonstrated improved sleep and reduced nighttime activity. Nocturnal eating ingestions admittedly were not reduced in this small study.[70] Among the author's series of patients with RLS, some early prospective data indicate that dopaminergic treatment results in a reduction (not an exacerbation) of nocturnal eating. Of the 8 RLS patients with nocturnal eating who had not yet been exposed to dopaminergic medications, 5 had resolution and 3 had improvement of nocturnal eating with dopaminergic therapy. Again, nocturnal eating symptoms demonstrated a clinical response parallel to that for motor RLS symptoms.[14] Finally, treatment with dopaminergic agents appears to improve other nonmotor manifestations of RLS. In particular, all of the patients who reported a remission of nocturnal smoking had been treated with dopaminergic agonists.[70]

Of importance, a substantial number of zolpidem-induced SRED cases are in the setting of patients with RLS.[28,35,39,42,56] As mentioned earlier, RLS is a condition distinct from, but often clinically confused with, PI. SRED, sleepwalking, and other complex sleep behaviors are rare (1% or less) in zolpidem-treated patients when RLS has been carefully excluded.[71–75] One report recognized a direct relationship between zolpidem-induced SRED and RLS. In this case both RLS

and nocturnal eating resolved once zolpidem was stopped and pramipexole (and clonazepam) was started. The same investigators reviewed 10 other cases and noted that in all 8 cases of zolpidem-related SRED in which RLS was subsequently considered, RLS was confirmed.[42] However, in a study of 19 patients with zolpidem-induced complex sleep behaviors, screening for RLS was notably absent.[41] In summary, the mistreatment of RLS as primary or conditioned insomnia may be a crucial underlying step in the pathogenesis of many amnestic SRED cases.

In conclusion, the following lines of evidence suggest that SRED may be characterized as a nonmotor manifestation of RLS, and that mistreatment of RLS as PI is a crucial step in the pathogenesis of drug-induced SRED cases. (1) RLS has frequently been described in cases of medication-induced and nonmedication-induced SRED. (2) Nocturnal eating is common in patients with RLS and was in fact reported in the original 1960 description by Ekbom. (3) SRED is common in patients with RLS. (4) The nocturnal eating in RLS is not merely "killing time" as patients with other causes of fragmented sleep, such as PI, rarely break the nighttime fast. (5) The compulsive nature of nocturnal eating in SRED is similar to the motor and other nonmotor manifestations of RLS. (6) PSG studies demonstrate periodic limb movements, RMMA, and bruxism in SRED. These phenomena are frequently noted in RLS, and like RLS are associated with dopaminergic dysfunction. (7) The nocturnal eating and motor restlessness of RLS frequently arise, intensify, and subside in parallel. (8) In several reports the underlying sleep fragmentation of drug-induced SRED was not caused by PI but instead by RLS, a common condition that is easily confused with (and treated as) PI. (9) The increase in amnestic SRED reports parallels the increase in benzodiazepine receptor agonist use. (10) The CNS actions of sedative-hypnotic

---

Box 1
Medications associated with SRED

Zolpidem immediate release

Zolpidem sustained release

Zopiclone

Zaleplon

Triazolam

Midazolam

Risperidone

Olanzapine

Table 3
Studies on pharmacotherapy for the treatment of SRED

Medication Class	Agent	Authors,[Ref.] Year	Study Design	Primary Diagnosis (No. of Subjects)	Results (Responders/Total Subjects)[a]
Dopaminergics	Carbidopa/levodopa	Schenck et al,[76] 1993	Case series	SRED (12)	(10/12) Temporary remission in 2/12
	Bromocriptine	Schenck et al,[76] 1993	Case series	SRED (3)	(2/3) Temporary remission in 1/3
	Pramipexole	Provini et al,[70] 2005	Pilot double-blind, placebo, crossover	SRED (11)	Decreased nocturnal activity as measured by actigraphy, no change in number of awakenings or ingestions
Antiseizure	Topiramate	Winkelman,[77] 2003	Open-label trial	SRED (2) NES (2)	(4/4) Mean weight loss 11.1 kg over 8.5 mo
	Topiramate	Martinez-Salio et al,[78] 2007	Case report	SRED (1)	(1/1) Two-year follow-up
	Topiramate	Schenck and Mahowald,[79] 2006	Case series	SRED (17)	(12/17) Mean weight loss of 9.2 kg among responders after 1.8 y
	Topiramate	Winkelman,[23] 2006	Open-label trial	SRED (25)	(17/25) Mean weight loss 11.1 kg over mean 11.6 mo; 21/25 adverse events, 7/17 responders discontinued after 1 y

[a] Responders are defined as those with elimination of nocturnal eating or diminished nocturnal eating along with other clinical improvement such as weight loss.

medications (suppression of memory and judgment) unleash predisposed behaviors, which in the case of RLS include inappropriate and amnestic ambulation with eating behavior. (11) Conversely, the incidence of SRED is rarely noted when patients have been rigorously evaluated and cases with underlying motor restlessness have been excluded from hypnotic treatment. (12) Finally, despite suggestions to the contrary, dopaminergic treatments for RLS appear to improve rather than exacerbate nocturnal eating and SRED.

TREATMENT

The first goal in treating dysfunctional nocturnal eating is to eliminate implicated medication (**Box 1**) and correct comorbid sleep disorders, especially RLS. The majority of patients with drug-induced SRED note improvement, if not outright resolution of nocturnal eating behavior after inducing agents are discontinued.[28,29,33–40] Rarely, patients who did not have nocturnal eating before exposure will have persisting episodes after cessation. It is not certain whether this is a temporary or persisting phenomena. Dopaminergics, opioids, and benzodiazepines are agents typically used in the treatment of RLS, and have been demonstrated to be effective in combined cases of RLS and SRED.[14,70,76] Of interest, SRED comorbid with sleepwalking can be effectively treated with these agents, suggesting the possibility of underlying motor restlessness as a cause of the patient's somnambulism (see earlier discussion). In one case series, 8 sleepwalking patients with SRED were effectively treated with bromocriptine and/or clonazepam.[76] In both reported cases of SRED with obstructive sleep apnea, continuous positive airway pressure eliminated both the sleep-disordered breathing and the nocturnal eating.[20]

At this time two classes of pharmacotherapy have been studied in SRED that appear to be potentially effective. In particular, dopaminergics, such as those used in RLS treatments, and the antiseizure medication topiramate have both demonstrated preliminary yet promising results. However, research on therapy for SRED is still in its infancy, and further investigations, in particular large randomized controlled trials, are necessary.

Dopaminergic agents are effective in the treatment of SRED even in the absence of known motor restlessness. The original case series noted that either bedtime levodopa or bromocriptine was effective in eliminating nocturnal eating.[76] Recently pramipexole, a dopamine agonist, was investigated in a small double-blind, placebo-controlled crossover trial. Pramipexole was well tolerated in all patients, including those without diagnosed RLS or periodic limb movement disorder. On pramipexole subjects noted improved sleep, and reduced nighttime activity was documented with actigraphy. There was no improvement in the number or duration of awakenings.[70] The main side effects of dopamine agonists include sedation, nausea, orthostasis, and impulsive behaviors.

Early studies indicate that the antiseizure medication topiramate may be an effective treatment for nocturnal eating in SRED. An open-label trial of topiramate in 4 patients with nocturnal eating demonstrated positive results. The agent was well tolerated, reports of nocturnal eating were diminished, and weight loss (mean of 11.1 kg) was noted in all 4 individuals over 8.5 months.[77] More recently, a 28-year-old obese man had a 10-year history of nocturnal eating episodes that were eliminated with topiramate. It was also reported that the agent was well tolerated over a 2-year follow-up.[78] In another case series, 12 of 17 SRED patients treated with topiramate were treatment responsive. The agent was well tolerated and over 1.8 years there was a mean weight loss of 9.2 kg among the treatment responders.[79] Another chart review of 25 follow-up SRED patients reported that 68% of SRED patients were treatment responders. Further, over 1 year 28% of patients lost more than 10% of their body weight. Adverse events were high, however, and 41% of patients discontinued the medication.[80] The main effects of topiramate include weight loss, paresthesias, renal calculus, cognitive dysfunction, and orthostasis. **Table 3** summarizes these findings.

SUMMARY

SRED occurs when there is a disruption of the nocturnal fast, with adverse consequences. Initial investigation should attempt to identify comorbid sleep disorders and to eliminate inducing agents. SRED is associated with psychotropic medication, most notably the BRA zolpidem, but with other sedative hypnotics as well. In particular, RLS is commonly associated with nocturnal eating, and treatment with dopaminergics often results in resolution of both conditions. PSG with a seizure montage at an accredited sleep laboratory is needed to identify and treat comorbid sleep disorders. At this time two types of pharmacotherapy, dopaminergics and the antiseizure agent topiramate, appear to be potentially effective. However, further therapeutic investigations of SRED are needed.

REFERENCES

1. Van Cauter E, Polonsky KS, Scheen AJ. Roles of circadian rhythmicity and sleep in human glucose regulation. Endocr Rev 1997;18(5):716–38.

2. Boyle PJ, Scott JC, Krentz AJ, et al. Diminished brain glucose metabolism is a significant determinant for falling rates of systemic glucose utilization during sleep in normal humans. J Clin Invest 1994; 93(2):529–35.

3. Maquet P, Dive D, Salmon E, et al. Cerebral glucose utilization during sleep-wake cycle in man determined by positron emission tomography and [^{18}F] 2-fluoro-2-deoxy-D-glucose method. Brain Res 1990;513(1):136–43.

4. Van Cauter E, Blackman JD, Roland D, et al. Modulation of glucose regulation and insulin secretion by circadian rhythmicity and sleep. J Clin Invest 1991; 88(3):934–42.

5. Van Cauter E, Spiegel K. Circadian and sleep control of endocrine secretions. In: Turek RW, See PC. Neurobiology of sleep and circadian rhythms. Marcel Dekker; 1999.

6. Holl RW, Hartman ML, Veldhuis JD, et al. Thirty-second sampling of plasma growth hormone in man: correlation with sleep stages. J Clin Endocrinol Metab 1991;72(4):854–61.

7. Simon C, Gronfier C, Schlienger JL, et al. Circadian and ultradian variations of leptin in normal man under continuous enteral nutrition: relationship to sleep and body temperature. J Clin Endocrinol Metab 1998;83(6):1893–9.

8. Dzaja A, Dalal MA, Himmerich H, et al. Sleep enhances nocturnal plasma ghrelin levels in healthy subjects. Am J Physiol Endocrinol Metab 2004;286(6):E963–7.

9. Schenck CH, Hurwitz TD, Bundlie SR, et al. Sleep-related eating disorders: polysomnographic correlates of a heterogeneous syndrome distinct from daytime eating disorders. Sleep 1991;14(5):419–31.

10. Winkelman JW. Clinical and polysomnographic features of sleep-related eating disorder. J Clin Psychiatry 1998;59(1):14–9.

11. American Academy of Sleep Medicine. In: Westchester IL, editor. International classification of sleep disorders: diagnostic and coding manual. 2nd edition. Westchester (IL): American Academy of Sleep Medicine; 2005. p. 173–6.

12. Stunkard AJ, Grace WJ, Wolff HG. The night-eating syndrome; a pattern of food intake among certain obese patients. Am J Med 1955;19(1):78–86.

13. Stunkard AJ, Allison KC, Lundgren JD, et al. A biobehavioural model of the night eating syndrome. Obes Rev 2009;10(Suppl 2):69–77.

14. Howell MJ, Schenck CH, Larson S, et al. Nocturnal eating and sleep-related eating disorder (SRED) are common among patients with restless legs syndrome. Sleep 2010;33:A227.

15. Provini F, Antelmi E, Vignatelli L, et al. Association of restless legs syndrome with nocturnal eating: a case-control study. Mov Disord 2009;24(6):871–7.

16. Lam SP, Fong SY, Yu MW, et al. Sleepwalking in psychiatric patients: comparison of childhood and adult onset. Aust N Z J Psychiatry 2009;43(5):426–30.

17. Vetrugno R, Manconi M, Ferini-Strambi L, et al. Nocturnal eating: sleep-related eating disorder or night eating syndrome? A videopolysomnographic study. Sleep 2006;29(7):949–54.

18. Winkelman JW, Herzog DB, Fava M. The prevalence of sleep-related eating disorder in psychiatric and non-psychiatric populations. Psychol Med 1999; 29(6):1461–6.

19. Lam SP, Fong SY, Ho CK, et al. Parasomnia among psychiatric outpatients: a clinical, epidemiologic, cross-sectional study. J Clin Psychiatry 2008;69(9): 1374–82.

20. Schenck CH, Mahowald MW. Review of nocturnal sleep-related eating disorders. Int J Eat Disord 1994;15(4):343–56.

21. Schenck CH. Paradox lost: midnight in the battleground of sleep and dreams. 1st edition. Minneapolis (MN): Extreme-Nights, LLC; 2006.

22. De Ocampo J, Foldvary N, Dinner DS, et al. Sleep-related eating disorder in fraternal twins. Sleep Med 2002;3(6):525–6.

23. Winkelman JW. Sleep-related eating disorder and night eating syndrome: sleep disorders, eating disorders, or both? Sleep 2006;29(7):876–7.

24. Nadel C. Somnambulism, bed-time medication and over-eating. Br J Psychiatry 1981;139:79.

25. Whyte J. Somnambulistic eating: a report of three cases. Int J Eat Disord 1990;9:577–81.

26. de Zwaan M, Roerig DB, Crosby RD, et al. Nighttime eating: a descriptive study. Int J Eat Disord 2006; 39(3):224–32.

27. Dolder CR, Nelson MH. Hypnosedative-induced complex behaviours: incidence, mechanisms and management. CNS Drugs 2008;22(12):1021–36.

28. Morgenthaler TI, Silber MH. Amnestic sleep-related eating disorder associated with zolpidem. Sleep Med 2002;3(4):323–7.

29. Schenck CH, Connoy DA, Castellanos M, et al. Zolpidem-induced sleep-related eating disorder (SRED) in 19 patients. Sleep 2005;28(Suppl):a259.

30. Paquet V, Strul J, Servais L, et al. Sleep-related eating disorder induced by olanzapine. J Clin Psychiatry 2002;63(7):597.

31. Lu ML, Shen WW. Sleep-related eating disorder induced by risperidone. J Clin Psychiatry 2004; 65(2):273–4.

32. Molina SM, Joshi KG. A case of zaleplon-induced amnestic sleep-related eating disorder. J Clin Psychiatry 2010;71(2):210–1.

33. Harazin J, Berigan TR. Zolpidem tartrate and somnambulism. Mil Med 1999;164(9):669–70.

34. Valiensi SM, Cristiano E, Martinez OA, et al. Sleep related eating disorders as a side effect of zolpidem. Medicina (B Aires) 2010;70(3):223–6 [in Spanish].

35. Sansone RA, Sansone LA. Zolpidem, somnambulism, and nocturnal eating. Gen Hosp Psychiatry 2008;30(1):90–1.

36. Dang A, Garg G, Rataboli PV. Zolpidem induced nocturnal sleep-related eating disorder (NSRED) in a male patient. Int J Eat Disord 2009;42(4): 385–6.

37. Wing YK, Lam SP, Li SX, et al. Sleep-related eating disorder and zolpidem: an open interventional cohort study. J Clin Psychiatry 2010;71(5):653–6.

38. Najjar M. Zolpidem and amnestic sleep related eating disorder. J Clin Sleep Med 2007;3(6):637–8.

39. Chiang A, Krystal A. Report of two cases where sleep related eating behavior occurred with the extended-release formulation but not the immediate-release formulation of a sedative-hypnotic agent. J Clin Sleep Med 2008;4(2):155–6.

40. Tsai MJ, Tsai YH, Huang YB. Compulsive activity and anterograde amnesia after zolpidem use. Clin Toxicol (Phila) 2007;45(2):179–81.

41. Hwang TJ, Ni HC, Chen HC, et al. Risk predictors for hypnosedative-related complex sleep behaviors: a retrospective, cross-sectional pilot study. J Clin Psychiatry 2010;71(10):1331–5.

42. Yun CH, Ji KH. Zolpidem-induced sleep-related eating disorder. J Neurol Sci 2010;288(1–2):200–1.

43. Hoque R, Chesson AL Jr. Zolpidem-induced sleepwalking, sleep related eating disorder, and sleep-driving: fluorine-18-flourodeoxyglucose positron emission tomography analysis, and a literature review of other unexpected clinical effects of zolpidem. J Clin Sleep Med 2009;5(5):471–6.

44. Gillin JC, Buchsbaum MS, Valladares-Neto DC, et al. Effects of zolpidem on local cerebral glucose metabolism during non-REM sleep in normal volunteers: a positron emission tomography study. Neuropsychopharmacology 1996;15(3):302–13.

45. Sanofi-Aventis 2005 financial report. Paris (France): Sanofi-Aventis; 2006.

46. Berger K, Luedemann J, Trenkwalder C, et al. Sex and the risk of restless legs syndrome in the general population. Arch Intern Med 2004;164(2):196–202.

47. Allen RP, Walters AS, Montplaisir J, et al. Restless legs syndrome prevalence and impact: REST general population study. Arch Intern Med 2005; 165(11):1286–92.

48. Ohayon MM, Guilleminault C, Priest RG. Night terrors, sleepwalking, and confusional arousals in the general population: their frequency and relationship to other sleep and mental disorders. J Clin Psychiatry 1999;60(4):268–76.

49. Paulus W, Dowling P, Rijsman R, et al. Update of the pathophysiology of the restless-legs-syndrome. Mov Disord 2007;22(Suppl 18):S431–9.

50. Bello NT, Hajnal A. Dopamine and binge eating behaviors. Pharmacol Biochem Behav 2010;97(1): 25–33.

51. Lavigne GJ, Kato T, Kolta A, et al. Neurobiological mechanisms involved in sleep bruxism. Crit Rev Oral Biol Med 2003;14(1):30–46.

52. Lavigne GJ, Montplaisir JY. Restless legs syndrome and sleep bruxism: prevalence and association among Canadians. Sleep 1994;17(8):739–43.

53. Manni R, Ratti MT, Tartara A. Nocturnal eating: prevalence and features in 120 insomniac referrals. Sleep 1997;20(9):734–8.

54. Satija P, Ondo WG. Restless legs syndrome: pathophysiology, diagnosis and treatment. CNS Drugs 2008;22(6):497–518.

55. Allen RP. Controversies and challenges in defining the etiology and pathophysiology of restless legs syndrome. Am J Med 2007;120(1 Suppl 1):S13–21.

56. Mahowald MW, Cramer Bornemann MA, Schenck CH. A case of reversible restless legs syndrome (RLS) and sleep-related eating disorder relapse triggered by acute right leg herpes zoster infection: literature review of spinal cord and peripheral nervous system contributions to RLS. Sleep Med 2010;11(6):583–5.

57. Maffettone C, De Martino L, Irace C, et al. Expression of iron-related proteins during infection by bovine herpes virus type-1. J Cell Biochem 2008; 104(1):213–23.

58. Walters AS. Toward a better definition of the restless legs syndrome. The International Restless Legs Syndrome Study Group. Mov Disord 1995;10(5): 634–42.

59. Provini F, Antelmi E, Vignatelli L, et al. Increased prevalence of nocturnal smoking in restless legs syndrome (RLS). Sleep Med 2010;11(2):218–20.

60. Picchietti D, Winkelman JW. Restless legs syndrome, periodic limb movements in sleep, and depression. Sleep 2005;28(7):891–8.

61. Winkelman JW, Finn L, Young T. Prevalence and correlates of restless legs syndrome symptoms in the Wisconsin Sleep Cohort. Sleep Med 2006;7(7): 545–52.

62. Lee HB, Hening WA, Allen RP, et al. Restless legs syndrome is associated with DSM-IV major depressive disorder and panic disorder in the community. Winter. J Neuropsychiatry Clin Neurosci 2008; 20(1):101–5.

63. International Restless Legs Syndrome Study Group. Restless legs syndrome or Ekbom's syndrome SLEEP. San Antonio (TX); 2010.

64. Nirenberg MJ, Waters C. Compulsive eating and weight gain related to dopamine agonist use. Mov Disord 2006;21(4):524–9.

65. Giladi N, Weitzman N, Schreiber S, et al. New onset heightened interest or drive for gambling, shopping, eating or sexual activity in patients with Parkinson's disease: the role of dopamine agonist treatment and

age at motor symptoms onset. J Psychopharmacol 2007;21(5):501–6.

66. Driver-Dunckley ED, Noble BN, Hentz JG, et al. Gambling and increased sexual desire with dopaminergic medications in restless legs syndrome. Clin Neuropharmacol 2007;30(5):249–55.

67. Tippmann-Peikert M, Park JG, Boeve BF, et al. Pathologic gambling in patients with restless legs syndrome treated with dopaminergic agonists. Neurology 2007;68(4):301–3.

68. Nirenberg MJ, Waters C. Nocturnal eating in restless legs syndrome. Mov Disord 2010;25(1):126–7.

69. Martin-Iverson MT, Dourish CT. Role of dopamine D-1 and D-2 receptor subtypes in mediating dopamine agonist effects on food consumption in rats. Psychopharmacology (Berl) 1988;96(3):370–4.

70. Provini F, Albani F, Vetrugno R, et al. A pilot double-blind placebo-controlled trial of low-dose pramipexole in sleep-related eating disorder. Eur J Neurol 2005;12(6):432–6.

71. Sauvanet JP, Maarek L, Roger M, et al. Open long-term trials with zolpidem in insomnia. In: Sauvanet JP, Langer SZ, Morselli PL, editors. Imidozopyridines in sleep disorders. New York: Raven Press; 1988. p. 339–49.

72. Roth T, Roehrs T, Vogel G. Zolpidem in the treatment of transient insomnia: a double-blind, randomized comparison with placebo. Sleep 1995;18(4):246–51.

73. Ganzoni E, Santoni JP, Chevillard V, et al. Zolpidem in insomnia: a 3-year post-marketing surveillance study in Switzerland. J Int Med Res 1995;23(1):61–73.

74. Holm KJ, Goa KL. Zolpidem: an update of its pharmacology, therapeutic efficacy and tolerability in the treatment of insomnia. Drugs 2000;59(4):865–89.

75. Roth T, Soubrane C, Titeux L, et al, Zoladult Study Group. Efficacy and safety of zolpidem-MR: a double-blind, placebo-controlled study in adults with primary insomnia. Sleep Med 2006;7(5):397–406.

76. Schenck CH, Hurwitz TD, O'Connor KA, et al. Additional categories of sleep-related eating disorders and the current status of treatment. Sleep 1993; 16(5):457–66.

77. Winkelman JW. Treatment of nocturnal eating syndrome and sleep-related eating disorder with topiramate. Sleep Med 2003;4(3):243–6.

78. Martinez-Salio A, Soler-Algarra S, Calvo-Garcia I, et al. Nocturnal sleep-related eating disorder that responds to topiramate. Rev Neurol 2007;45(5): 276–9.

79. Schenck CH, Mahowald MW. Topiramate therapy of sleep related eating disorder (SRED). Sleep 2006; 29:a268.

80. Winkelman JW. Efficacy and tolerability of open-label topiramate in the treatment of sleep-related eating disorder: a retrospective case series. J Clin Psychiatry 2006;67(11):1729–34.

Sleep and Drug-Impaired Driving Overlap Syndrome

Mark R. Pressman, PhD, D.ABSM[a,b,c,*]

KEYWORDS

- Zolpidem • Sleep driving • Sleepwalking • CNS
- NREM parasomnia • Residual drug effect

Driving while under the influence of zolpidem, zopiclone, and other sedative/hypnotics has been called sleep driving (R v. Lowe, 2005 in Manchester, UK, unpublished legal case).[1–3] Sleep driving is most often described as a variant of sleepwalking, along with sleep eating,[4] sleep sex,[5] and sleep violence.[6–8] Sleepwalking is a well-described sleep disorder that occurs following a partial arousal from deep sleep, usually within the first 2 hours of sleep. It is not related to dreaming or prior psychological trauma.[9,10] However, a recent review of the sleep-driving research concluded that most impaired driving labeled as sleep driving was instead related to misuse or abuse of sedative/hypnotics, in particular zolpidem and zopiclone.[11] Only 18 cases of impaired driving attributed to underlying sleepwalking pathophysiology were identified.[1,2,4,12]

Sleepwalking and its variants are diagnosed based on clinical history.[13] There are no generally accepted sleep laboratory findings or other reliable biomarkers, and these are not required for diagnosis.[14] Only 2 of these 18 cases provided any clinical history supportive of sleepwalking, and these histories are much more limited than typically required.[1,12] Further, these published cases do not provide a detailed description of behavior before, during, and after the impaired-driving episode so that the context along with priming and triggering factors can be determined

and understood. Rather, the case histories of impaired drivers attributed to sleepwalking and those attributed to the effects of sedative/hypnotic drugs only provide descriptions of driver signs, symptoms, and behaviors at the time of arrest and during sobriety testing by the arresting officer.[15–18]

Impaired driving associated with zolpidem and zopiclone has been reported to result from significant drug levels present in a waking and driving individual. This drug level, while awake, can result if the sedative/hypnotic (1) is taken at the wrong time of day, (2) is taken at higher than the recommended doses, (3) is taken concomitantly with central nervous system (CNS) depressants, or (4) is caused by a failure to allow sufficient sleep time or time in bed.[19] Many impaired drivers in these cases were able to respond to police officer questions and requests but were unable to complete sobriety testing because they were unable to stand up and maintain balance safely.[16] This pattern differs from the typical sleepwalker who, in most cases, can stand up and walk safely but whose higher cognitive functions are essentially absent. Because of the severe cognitive impairment, sleepwalkers would not be able to interact with police officers or even understand what was being asked of them. A sudden confrontation by a police officer might provoke violent, defensive behavior in a sleepwalker. A recent

The author has nothing to disclose.
a Sleep Medicine Services, The Lankenau Medical Center and Lankenau Institute for Medical Research, 100 Lancaster Avenue, Wynnewood, PA 19096, USA
b Department of Medicine, Jefferson Medical College, Walnut Street, Philadelphia, PA 19107, USA
c Villanova School of Law, 299 North Spring Mill Road, Villanova, PA 19085, USA
* Corresponding author. Sleep Medicine Services, The Lankenau Medical Center and Lankenau Institute for Medical Research, 100 Lancaster Avenue, Wynnewood, PA 19096.
E-mail address: sleepwake@comcast.net

Sleep Med Clin 6 (2011) 441–445
doi:10.1016/j.jsmc.2011.08.003

review of sleep driving suggested the progression of symptoms in sleep driving is suggestive of an overlap syndrome.[11] In this overlap syndrome, sleep driving would be initiated because of a sudden arousal from deep sleep, as is typical of sleepwalking. The sedative/hypnotic drug may play a role in preventing full wakefulness. However, once the sleepwalking episode that initiated the behavior ended, typically in minutes, the driving episode would continue because significant blood levels of the zolpidem, zopiclone, or other sedative/hypnotic drug would remain active causing CNS depression.

The first case of apparent zolpidem-associated sleep driving with a detailed description of the complex behaviors before, during, and after the episode, along with personal and family sleep history, is presented. Evidence in support of a sleep and drug-impaired driving overlap syndrome is discussed.

CASE REPORT

In the spring of 2009, Mr EP was arrested for driving under the influence of zolpidem in a small city in the Northeast United States. At the time, EP was 21 years old, a recent college graduate, and varsity athlete. He was healthy with no major medical or psychiatric complaints other than difficulty falling asleep. EP reported he had severe difficulty falling asleep until 3 to 4 AM during his last 2 years of college. A clinical interview revealed that once asleep, he was able to sleep normally and awaken refreshed. Along with the absence of signs and symptoms of other sleep disorders, his complaint was most consistent with the diagnosis of a biologic rhythm disorder common in college students: delayed sleep phase syndrome (DSPS).[20] His sleep problems were further exacerbated by the requirement of athletic practices starting at 6 AM. To make up for the insufficient nighttime sleep, he would nap once or twice later in the day. This practice resulted in a polyphasic sleep schedule. After complaining to his physician of insomnia, he was prescribed zolpidem 12.5 mg (CR formulation) at bedtime. He found that the medication did assist him in falling asleep faster, although it did not eliminate his insomnia completely. Persistence of the sleep complaint would be expected because sedative/hypnotics are not a cure for DSPS.

EP routinely drank 1 to 2 glasses of port or other alcoholic beverage in the evening 30 to 60 minutes before taking zolpidem. He had followed this pattern for almost 2 years without any adverse effects. He stated his physician had not warned against using alcohol. He had not read the package insert. However, there was a label on his pill bottle stating, "do not take with alcohol." EP related that he assumed this meant taking alcohol and zolpidem at the same time might result in deeper or longer sleep. He was not aware of the risk that zolpidem alone, or in combination with alcohol, may result in complex behaviors.

Personal and Family Sleep History

According to both friends and family, EP had a life-long history of sleepwalking and similar behaviors. EP's father described episodes of sleepwalking occurring at least weekly during childhood and persisting into his teenage years. Sleepwalking episodes would typically occur 1 to 2 hours after bedtime and involve EP leaving the bedroom and wandering about the house, along with other complex and sometimes bizarre behaviors. EP had to be restrained from leaving the family home on more than one occasion. Family and friends reported EP to have been unresponsive and amnestic from these episodes the next morning. None of these episodes were related to alcohol or sedative/hypnotic use.

There were 2 prior sleepwalking episodes that might have been related to either alcohol or zolpidem. The first occurred approximately 2 years before the current episode. The campus police found EP wandering around the college grounds wearing boxer shorts and 2 robes in the middle of the night. He does not recall if alcohol was involved, but thinks he had taken zolpidem. He has no memory of this episode. Cumulative partial sleep deprivation may have been a priming factor.

The second episode occurred while visiting friends during the Christmas holiday. EP flew from coast to coast and arrived jet-lagged. EP went to sleep approximately 3 hours after dinner, which did include alcohol. Approximately 1 hour later, his friends, who had not yet gone to sleep, heard yelling and noise from an adjacent room. They found EP had climbed on top of a combination washer/dryer and somehow inserted himself into the 2-ft opening between the machine and the ceiling. They tried to coax him down. They described him as confrontational and confused. Eventually, he did climb down; but when approached to lead him back to bed, he became agitated and fearful. He was eventually led back to bed and had no memory of this episode in the morning. The episode occurred before he had started taking zolpidem and he denied drinking alcohol excessively 3 hours earlier. Severe sleep deprivation related to his jet lag may have been a priming factor.

There is also a strong family history of sleep-walking. EP's sister suffered from frequent episodes of sleepwalking and on several occasions left their home in her pajamas.

EP has a strong history of sleepwalking behaviors persisting to the present. These behaviors are consistent with diagnostic criteria: (1) most often occurred 1 to 4 hours after sleep onset, (2) involved wandering or odd behaviors with eyes open, (3) was unresponsive to others, (4) agitated when confronted, (5) amnesic the next morning, (6) associated with sleep deprivation, and (7) had a familial pattern.

Chronology of Current Episode

- 11:15 PM (approximate): While watching TV with his roommate, EP is reported to have had 1 to 2 glasses of port.
- 11:45 PM (approximate): EP took his usual dose of zolpidem 12.5 mg just before lights out as witnessed by his roommate. Lights were then turned out, the covers pulled up, and the door closed. EP seemed to his roommate to have "gone to sleep." He went to sleep wearing boxer shorts.
- 11:45 PM to 1:50 AM: EP apparently partially arouses from a deep sleep.
  - Gets out of bed in sleepwalking state
  - Puts on clothing he would not typically wear
  - Takes keys and wallet and leaves apartment
  - Goes to car, opens door, and gets in
  - Puts key in ignition and starts car
  - Drives 2.5 miles to area he is not familiar with
  - Stops car in middle of intersection (responded to red light too late?).

Chronology from here on is based primarily on police reports.

- 1:50 AM: The police report filed by patrol officer P indicates he came to a car stopped in the middle of an intersection while the light was red.
- When the traffic light turned green, the car began to move forward.
- Patrol officer P turned on the emergency lights and siren.
- The car driver pulled to the left.
- The car pulled up on the curb, then back on the roadway, stopping.
- Patrol officer P asked the driver for his license and registration.
- The driver produced, with "great difficulty and effort," the license only.

- The patrol officer questioned the driver as to why he had stopped in the middle of the intersection.
- In "extremely slow speech," the driver answered, "huh, what are you talking about?"
- The driver denied hitting the curb.
- The odor of alcohol was detected.
- The driver stated he had been drinking earlier.
- The driver had difficulty exiting the car.
- The driver exited the car and had to hold onto the parking meter to stop from falling over.
- Sobriety testing occurred:
  - Successfully repeated alphabet, but it was "slow and slurred"
  - Finger-to-nose test: successful 2 of 4 times, but was very unsteady standing
  - Heel to toe: failed, unable to walk the 10 required steps
  - Tests stopped out of concern for driver's safety
- He was placed under arrest and put in handcuffs.
- 2:20 AM: He was returned to the police station booking desk.
- The breath alcohol testing revealed a blood alcohol level of 0.05.
- On further questioning by the police, EP stated he had taken zolpidem before bedtime.
- He was placed under arrest for operating under the influence.
- Blood testing for zolpidem levels was not performed.
- He stayed in lockup until the next morning.
- On awakening, EP had no memory of where he was, how he got there, or what had happened the night before.

DISCUSSION

The case of EP seems typical of previously described cases of impaired driving associated with zolpidem use. His behaviors closely follow those of many reported cases of driving under the influence (DUI) associated with zolpidem and other sedative/hypnotics. However, previously published case reports generally started and ended with the impaired driving portion of the episode and give no hint as to how the driver came to be in a moving vehicle.[2,16,18,21] However, this case provides details as to how this episode started and additional details, especially regarding prior and current sleep history and the context and circumstances of the episode. The current case report starts with a series of complex behaviors in sleep that are consistent with sleepwalking. These occurred approximately 2 hours after bedtime consistent with an arousal from deep sleep that is typical of a non–rapid eye movement (NREM) parasomnia.[10] Thus, the driving episode was likely to have begun while in the middle of a sleepwalking-related state. Many behaviors performed during sleepwalking and its variants are considered to be automatic in that they can be performed with little or no conscious awareness.[22] In this case, EP had probably performed the driving-related behaviors thousands of times before. As in many NREM parasomnias, saying a behavior is automatic does not necessarily mean this behavior was performed correctly. EP dressed, but he did not put on clothing typical for him. EP drove a car, but he went to an area he was unfamiliar with. EP tried to stop for a red light, but he actually stopped in the middle of an intersection. EP pulled over when signaled by the police, but he pulled off the road in the wrong direction and onto the curb and sidewalk. EP also had amnesia for the episode, typical of NREM parasomnias.

Only after entering the car does the sleep-driving portion of the episode begin. Although this case of sleep driving clearly began as a complex sleepwalking episode, the description of the end of the episode features behaviors that were not typical of sleepwalking and other NREM parasomnias unrelated to drugs or medications. EP was likely awakened by the sound of the police siren or by the police themselves. As described by the police, EP seemed severely physically impaired, so much so that he could not complete sobriety testing. He was unable to stand up unaided, but nevertheless was able to respond, albeit very sluggishly and poorly, to requests to see his drivers license. He did not awaken fully and did not act aggressively toward the police officers. This type of behavior has been reported in cases of zolpidem-impaired driving, most likely caused by misuse or abuse, but is not typical of sleepwalking episodes.[11] These behaviors have more in common with general CNS depression and include many of the same characteristics that have been reported in other zolpidem-impaired drivers.

There are 4 possible scenarios that could account for EP's behaviors. The first possibility is that the presence of zolpidem extended the sleep-driving episode by interacting with the deep sleep or EP's genetic predisposition for sleepwalking. The second possibility is that the underlying sleepwalking episodes ended, but the typical transitional period of confusion at the end of sleepwalking episodes was extended or exacerbated by the presence of zolpidem. The third possibility is that the police failed to awaken EP completely because of CNS depression or sleep inertia.[23] The fourth possibility, and the one most consistent with published scientific data, is that once awakened by the police, he had attempted to respond and perform sobriety testing in the presence of a residual but high blood level of zolpidem.[24] Numerous experimental studies have been conducted in which normal subjects were awakened from sleep 2 to 4 hours after taking a sedative/hypnotic.[25,26] The behaviors after the experimental awakening closely resembled EP's in this case and other drivers stopped for a zolpidem-associated DUI. However, most experimental studies were not monitored concurrently by polysomnography (sleep studies); thus, it is not known if these subjects were awakened out of deep sleep. Depression of arousal by zolpidem or alcohol may have produced a similar effect to that of sleep deprivation.[27] Nevertheless, an incomplete arousal from sleep would seem to be necessary to trigger and produce EP's sleepwalking and sleep-driving behaviors. The actual trigger is not known in this case.

In summary, sleep driving properly refers to a series of complex behaviors occurring out of deep sleep and should not be confused with impaired driving solely caused by misuse or abuse of zolpidem or other sedative/hypnotics. However, sleepwalking and drug effects may overlap. EP's episode consisted of a series of complex sleepwalking behaviors that included sleep driving. However, his behavior, once the police intervened, did not resemble the behaviors of a sleepwalker in which physical function is only slightly impaired, whereas higher cognitive function (memory, planning, social interaction) is severely impaired or absent. Rather, his behavior as reported by the police was most consistent with drug-induced CNS depression affecting both physical and mental abilities severely and equally. It seems likely that once the NREM parasomnia or underlying period of deep sleep ended, the longer-acting residual effects of the zolpidem persisted, directly impairing wakefulness. Thus, these driving behaviors are likely the product of both sleepwalking pathophysiology and the residual effects of zolpidem. These 2 factors combine to produce a sleep and drug-impaired driving overlap syndrome.

REFERENCES

1. Doane JA, Dalpiaz AS. Zolpidem-induced sleep-driving. Am J Med 2008;121(11):e5.
2. Southworth MR, Kortepeter C, Hughes A. Nonbenzodiazepine hypnotic use and cases of "sleep driving". Ann Intern Med 2008;148(6):486–7.

3. FDA requests label change for all sleep disorder drug products. Washington, DC: FDA; March 14, 2007.

4. Schenck C, Connoy D, Castellanos M, et al. Zolpidem induced amnestic sleep-related eating disorder (SRED) in 19 patients [abstract]. Sleep 2005;28(Suppl):A259.

5. Guilleminault C, Moscovitch A, Yuen K, et al. Atypical sexual behavior during sleep. Psychosom Med 2002;64(2):328–36.

6. Broughton RJ, Shimizu T. Sleep-related violence: a medical and forensic challenge. Sleep 1995; 18(9):727–30.

7. Pressman MR. Disorders of arousal from sleep and violent behavior: the role of physical contact and proximity. Sleep 2007;30(8):1039–47.

8. Broughton R, Billings R, Cartwright R, et al. Homicidal somnambulism: a case report. Sleep 1994; 17(3):253–64.

9. Broughton RJ. Sleep disorders: disorders of arousal? Enuresis, somnambulism, and nightmares occur in confusional states of arousal, not in "dreaming sleep". Science 1968;159(819):1070–8.

10. Mahowald MW, Cramer Bornemann M. Non-REM parasomnias. In: Kryger MH, Roth C, Dement WC, editors. Principles and practice of sleep medicine. 5th edition. Philadelphia: Elsevier Saunders; 2011. p. 1075–82.

11. Pressman MR. Sleep Driving and Z-Drugs: sleepwalking variant or misuse of drugs? Sleep Med Rev 2011;15:285–92.

12. Hoque R, Chesson AL Jr. Zolpidem-induced sleepwalking, sleep related eating disorder, and sleep-driving: fluorine-18-flourodeoxyglucose positron emission tomography analysis, and a literature review of other unexpected clinical effects of zolpidem. J Clin Sleep Med 2009;5(5):471–6.

13. American Academy of Sleep Medicine. ICSD-2-International Classification of Sleep Disorders. diagnostic and coding manual. 2nd edition. Westchester (IL): American Academy of Sleep Medicine; 2005.

14. Pressman MR. Factors that predispose, prime and precipitate NREM parasomnias in adults: clinical and forensic implications. Sleep Med Rev 2007; 11(1):5–30.

15. Meeker JE, Baselt RC. Six cases of impaired driving following recent use of the sleep inducer zolpidem (Ambien) [abstract]. American Academy of Forensic Sciences Annual Meeting. Nashville, 1996.

16. Logan BK, Couper FJ. Zolpidem and driving impairment. J Forensic Sci 2001;46(1):105–10.

17. Johnson EO, Roehrs T, Roth T, et al. Epidemiology of alcohol and medication as aids to sleep in early adulthood. Sleep 1998;21(2):178–86.

18. Liddicoat LJ, Harding P. Ambien: drives like a dream: case studies of zolpidem impaired drivers in Wisconsin. 58th meeting American Academy of Forensic Sciences. Februay 23, 2006.

19. Verster JC, Volkerts ER, Olivier B, et al. Zolpidem and traffic safety - the importance of treatment compliance. Curr Drug Saf 2007;2(3):220–6.

20. Weitzman ED, Czeisler CA, Coleman RM, et al. Delayed sleep phase syndrome. A chronobiological disorder with sleep-onset insomnia. Arch Gen Psychiatry 1981;38(7):737–46.

21. Johnson WR, Cochems AK, et al. Zolpidem impaired drivers in Wisconsin: a six year retrospective Wisconsin state laboratory of hygiene. Madison (WI): Society of Forensic Toxicology; 2005.

22. Cramer Bornemann M, Mahowald MW. Sleep Forensics. In: Kryger MH, Roth C, Dement WC, editors. Principles and Practice of Sleep Medicine. 5th edition. Philadelphia: Elsevier Saunders; 2011. p. 725–33.

23. Wertz AT, Ronda JM, Czeisler CA, et al. Effects of sleep inertia on cognition. JAMA 2006;295(2):163–4.

24. Frey DJ, Ortega JD, Wiseman C, et al. Influence of zolpidem and sleep inertia on balance and cognition during nighttime awakening: a randomized placebo-controlled trial. J Am Geriatr Soc 2011;59(1):73–81.

25. Verster JC, Volkerts ER, Schreuder AH, et al. Residual effects of middle-of-the-night administration of zaleplon and zolpidem on driving ability, memory functions, and psychomotor performance. J Clin Psychopharmacol 2002;22(6):576–83.

26. Verster JC, Veldhuijzen DS, Patat A, et al. Hypnotics and driving safety: meta-analyses of randomized controlled trials applying the on-the-road driving test. Curr Drug Saf 2006;1(1):63–71.

27. Pilon M, Montplaisir J, Zadra A. Precipitating factors of somnambulism: impact of sleep deprivation and forced arousals. Neurology 2008;70:2284–90.

Non–Rapid Eye Movement Parasomnias: Diagnostic Methods

Antonio Zadra, PhD[a,b,]*, Mathieu Pilon, PhD[b,c]

KEYWORDS

- NREM parasomnias • Sleepwalking • Somnambulism
- Sleep terrors • Diagnostic assessment

The American Academy of Sleep Medicine's *International Classification of Sleep Disorders (ICSD-II)*[1] defines parasomnias as "undesirable physical events or experiences that occur during entry into sleep, within sleep or during arousals from sleep." Depending on their exact manifestations, frequency, and intensity, parasomnias can be considered normal sleep phenomena and may not significantly affect sleep quality or quantity or daytime functioning. In some cases, however, episodes can lead to self-injuries, psychological distress, and sleep disruption, thereby seriously affecting the patient as well as family members.

Parasomnias are classified into 3 categories: (1) parasomnias associated with non–rapid eye movement (NREM) sleep (eg, sleepwalking and sleep terrors), (2) parasomnias associated with rapid eye movement (REM) sleep (eg, nightmare disorder and REM sleep behavior disorder [RBD]), and (3) other parasomnias (eg, sleep enuresis and sleep-related groaning). This article focuses on diagnostic considerations of 2 prototypic NREM sleep parasomnias, namely, sleepwalking (somnambulism) and sleep terrors. Together with confusional arousals, sleepwalking and sleep terrors are collectively termed disorders of arousal[2] because of the autonomic and motor arousal that drives the patient toward a state of partial wakefulness from sleep. A summary and comparison of the main features of NREM and REM sleep parasomnias are presented in **Table 1**.

Although disorders of arousal vary along dimensions of emotional, autonomic, and motor activation, they nevertheless share several characteristics. NREM parasomnias are common in children and tend to decrease in frequency with age. Episodes generally arise out of slow wave sleep (SWS; stages 3 and 4 of NREM sleep) and, more rarely, from stage 2 sleep. As a consequence, NREM parasomnias tend to take place in the first third of the night when SWS is predominant. Symptoms and manifestations of disorders of arousal can be considered along a spectrum, but most episodes are characterized by misperception and relative unresponsiveness to external stimuli, mental confusion, automatic behaviors, perceived threat, and variable retrograde amnesia. Conditions that intensify sleep, such as intense physical activity, hyperthyroidism, fever, sleep deprivation, and neuroleptics or medications with depressive central nervous system effects, can facilitate or precipitate NREM parasomnias in predisposed individuals. Factors that fragment sleep, including sleep-disordered breathing, periodic leg movement syndrome, stress, and environmental or endogenous stimuli can have similar effects. A common genetic component is suspected because a positive family history is often reported by

This work was supported by a grant from the Canadian Institutes of Health Research (CIHR).

a Department of Psychology, Université de Montréal, C.P. 6128, Succursale Centre-ville, Montreal, Québec H3C 3J7, Canada
b Center for Advanced Research in Sleep Medicine, Hôpital du Sacré-Cœur, 5400 Boul. Gouin Ouest, Montréal, Québec H4J 1C5, Canada
c Ste-Justine Hospital Research Center, 3175 chemin Côte Ste-Catherine, Montréal, Québec H3T 1C5, Canada
* Corresponding author. Department of Psychology, Université de Montréal, C.P. 6128, Succursale Centre-ville, Montreal, Québec H3C 3J7, Canada.
E-mail address: antonio.zadra@umontreal.ca

Sleep Med Clin 6 (2011) 447–458
doi:10.1016/j.jsmc.2011.08.001

Table 1
Comparison of common features of NREM and REM sleep parasomnias

	Confusional Arousal	Somnambulism	Sleep Terrors	Nightmares	RBD
Time of night	First third to half of the sleep period	First third to half of the sleep period	First third to half of the sleep period	Last half of the sleep period	Last half of the sleep period
Sleep stage	SWS	SWS	SWS	REM	REM without atonia
Associated activity	May sit up in bed	Simple to complex movements. Possible ambulation	Sits, screams. Agitated motor activity	Movements are rare and limited	Behavior that correlates with dream content
Duration	1–15 min	1–30 min	1–10 min	3–20 min	1–10 min
Autonomic activation	Low	Low to moderate	Moderate to extreme	None to moderate	Low to moderate
Recall for the event	Variable amnesia for the event	Variable amnesia for the event	Variable amnesia for the event	Vivid and detailed dream recall	Vivid and detailed dream recall
Full awakening	Uncommon	Uncommon	Uncommon	Common	Common
State after event	Confused/disoriented	Confused/disoriented	Confused/disoriented	Fully awake and functional	Fully awake and functional
Arousal threshold	High	High	High	Low	Low
Reduced in sleep laboratory	Yes	Yes	Yes	Yes	No
PSG findings	Partial arousals from SWS	Partial arousals from SWS	Partial arousals from SWS	REM	Excessive EMG activity during REM
Potential for injury/ violence	Yes	Yes	Yes	No	Yes

Abbreviations: EMG, electromyography; PSG, polysomnography; SWS, slow wave sleep.

people with an arousal disorder.[3,4] HLA-DQB1 typing in sleepwalkers and their families indicates that somnambulism may be associated with excessive transmission of the HLA-DQB1*05 and *04 alleles.[5] The genetic locus of sleepwalking was recently linked to chromosome 20q12-q13.12 in a 4-generation family study.[6]

The occurrence of NREM parasomnias in children is frequently viewed as a relatively benign and common event that resolves spontaneously. In adults, however, these disorders often pose greater problems, including psychological distress and apprehension, social inconveniences, and serious sleep-related injury to the sleeper or others. Injurious NREM sleep parasomnias in adults are particularly well documented.[7–9]

Establishing a correct diagnosis for NREM parasomnias is vital for the patient's proper treatment as well as in light of the growing number of medicolegal cases of sleep-related violence. Unlike most sleep disorders, the diagnosis of NREM parasomnias is often made primarily or exclusively on the basis of the patient's detailed history, including complete description of the time course and content of sleep-related behaviors. Descriptive information from family members or a bed partner and the use of home video recording (preferably with an infrared vision–enabled video camera) can be particularly valuable in further characterizing behavioral manifestations. Diagnostic assessments, however, can be complicated by several mediating factors, including poor or nonexistent recall of episodes, a history of unusually violent or injurious sleep-related behaviors, presence of excessive daytime sleepiness, associated medical or neurologic conditions, and the lack of validated sleep protocols to directly confirm the diagnosis.

The clinical criteria for sleepwalking and sleep terrors in the American Psychiatric Association's *Diagnostic and Statistical Manual of Mental Disorders* (Fourth Edition [*DSM-IV*])[10] and the American Academy of Sleep Medicine's *ICSD-II*[1] are presented in **Box 1**. Key assessment issues that should be covered during the clinical history for somnambulism and sleep terrors are presented in **Box 2**. In the following sections, important dimensions and tools related to the diagnosis of sleepwalking and sleep terrors are reviewed. These dimensions and tools include clinical presentation, phenomenological considerations, psychological testing, polysomnography, daytime functioning, brain imaging, and differential diagnosis.

CLINICAL PRESENTATION

The symptoms and manifestations that characterize NREM parasomnias can vary considerably both within and across patients. A sleepwalker's emotional expression can range from neutral or calm to extremely agitated while actual physical behaviors can range from simple actions (eg, sitting up in bed, mumbling, fingering bed sheets) to complex behaviors (eg, rearranging furniture, inappropriate sexual activity, playing a musical instrument, driving an automobile). The sleepwalker's eyes are usually open throughout an episode, and the sleepwalker may spontaneously return to bed or eventually lie down to sleep elsewhere. Given the heterogeneous nature of sleepwalking episodes, their duration can vary from a few seconds to dozens of minutes. Moreover, an episode can be composed of 2 overlapping disorders such as a sleep terror followed by sleepwalking. In more extreme cases, exhibited behaviors can include driving motor vehicles, inappropriate sexual activity, suspected suicide, and even homicide and attempted homicide, thereby raising vital questions as to the medicoforensic implications of these acts.[11]

Patients suffering from sleep terrors (also known as night terrors or pavor nocturnus) also experience arousals from SWS but typically scream loudly, sit up in bed with a panic-stricken expression, and show other autonomic nervous system manifestations of intense fear. These manifestations may include sweating, flushing of the skin, mydriasis, tachycardia, and rapid breathing. The episodes, which typically occur within 90 minutes after sleep onset, can include more complex behavioral manifestations, such as leaving the bed, fleeing the room, or thrashing around. These more extreme episodes can result in self-injuries, property damage, and considerable distress in family members of affected patients. Sleep terrors tend to be of short duration, often from less than a minute to a few minutes, but they can also be complex and co-occur with sleepwalking, making the differentiation between these 2 NREM parasomnias ambiguous and difficult. Inconsolability is a key feature of sleep terrors, and attempting to console or awaken an individual during a sleep terror can prolong or intensify the episode. Once the sleep terror episode has subsided, the person usually does not fully awaken, returns to sleep, and remains partially or completely amnesic for the event the following day.

PHENOMENOLOGICAL INQUIRY AND EPISODE RECALL

Both the *DSM* and *ICSD* diagnostic criteria for sleepwalking and sleep terrors include experiencing complete or partial amnesia for the episode. Although disorders of arousal are often characterized in terms of their automatic behaviors and

Box 1
Clinical criteria for sleepwalking and sleep terror disorder

DSM-IV diagnostic criteria for sleepwalking disorder (307.46)

1. Repeated episodes of rising from bed during sleep and walking about occur, usually during the first third of the major sleep episode.

2. While sleepwalking, the person has a blank staring face, is relatively unresponsive to the efforts of others to communicate with him or her, and can be awakened only with great difficulty.

3. On awakening (either from the sleepwalking episode or the next morning), the person has amnesia for the episode.

4. Within several minutes after awakening from the sleepwalking episode, there is no impairment of mental activity or behavior (although there may initially be a short period of confusion or disorientation).

5. The sleepwalking causes clinically significant distress or impairment in social, occupational, or other important areas of functioning.

6. The disturbance is not because of the direct physiologic effects of a substance (eg, a drug of abuse, a medication) or a general medical condition.

ICSD-II diagnostic criteria for sleepwalking disorder

1. Ambulation occurs during sleep.

2. Persistence of sleep, an altered state of consciousness, or impaired judgment during ambulation demonstrated by at least 1 of the following:

   a. Difficulty in arousing the person

   b. Mental confusion when awakened from an episode

   c. Amnesia (complete or partial) for the episode

   d. Routine behaviors that occur at inappropriate times

   e. Inappropriate or nonsensical behaviors

   f. Dangerous or potentially dangerous behaviors

3. The disturbance is not better explained by another sleep disorder, medical or neurologic disorder, mental disorder, medication use, or substance use disorder.

DSM-IV diagnostic criteria for sleep terror disorder (307.46)

1. Recurrent episodes of abrupt awakening from sleep occur, usually during the first third of the major sleep episode and beginning with a panicky scream.

2. Intense fear and signs of autonomic arousal, such as tachycardia, rapid breathing, and sweating, during each episode.

3. Relative unresponsiveness to efforts of others to comfort the person during the episode.

4. No detailed dream is recalled, and there is amnesia for the episode.

5. The episodes cause clinically significant distress or impairment in social, occupational, or other important areas of functioning.

6. The disturbance is not because of the direct physiologic effects of a substance (eg, a drug of abuse, a medication) or a general medical condition.

ICSD-II diagnostic criteria for sleep terror disorder

1. A sudden episode of terror occurs during sleep, usually initiated by a cry or loud scream that is accompanied by autonomic nervous system and behavioral manifestations of intense fear.

2. At least 1 of the following associated features is present:

   a. Difficulty in arousing the person

   b. Mental confusion when awakened from an episode

   c. Amnesia (complete or partial) for the episode

   d. Dangerous or potentially dangerous behaviors

3. The disturbance is not better explained by another sleep disorder, medical or neurologic disorder, mental disorder, medication use, or substance use disorder.

Data from APA. Diagnostic and statistical manual of mental disorders: DSM-IV. 4th edition. Washington, DC: American Psychiatric Association; 1994; and ICSD-II, International Classification of Sleep Disorders. 2nd edition.

Box 2
Key assessment features during a clinical interview for NREM parasomnias

- Age of onset
- Timing of the episode during the sleep period
- Episode frequency and duration
- Detailed description of the episode, including behavioral manifestations, effect, and mentation during and after the event
- Responsiveness to external stimuli during the event
- Level of consciousness or awareness when awakened from an episode
- Memory for the event
- Precipitating or triggering factors
- Sleep-wake pattern and sleep environment
- Symptoms of daytime sleepiness
- Symptoms of other sleep disorders
- Familial history for NREM parasomnias and other sleep disorders
- Medical, psychiatric, and neurologic history
- Medication and substance use

retrograde amnesia, recent work indicates that perceptual, cognitive, and affective dimensions can play an important role in the subjective experience of adult sleepwalking. The discrepancy between the detailed phenomenological contents sometimes recalled by patients and current diagnostic criteria for episode amnesia often poses a problem to clinicians and contributes low interobserver reliability for the final diagnosis of sleepwalking.[12] One questionnaire-based study[13] of 68 adult patients consecutively referred to a sleep disorders clinic for chronic sleepwalking found that perceptual elements from the sleeper's actual environment during somnambulistic episodes were sometimes (25%), often (37%), or always (16%) recalled. In this study, 47 patients (69%) reported that various forms of mental content or sleep mentation (eg, images, thoughts, emotions) often or always accompanied their episodes. Furthermore, the displayed behaviors were construed by most patients as being motivated by an intrinsic sense of urgency or underlying reason that accounts for their actions during actual episodes. More recently, a study of patients with somnambulism/sleep terrors[14] showed that more than 70% of participants report experiencing sleep mentation during their episodes.

Similarly, laboratory investigations of adult sleepwalkers suggest that when available, patients'

phenomenological contents are broadly consistent with the observed behaviors during an episode. For instance, as part of a study on the use of forced arousals from auditory stimuli to experimentally induce somnambulistic events,[15] 1 patient experienced an episode during which he quickly removed his pillow and frantically examined the back of his bed. The patient, who had recently become a dad, later reported that he believed his newborn had fallen behind the bed. Another patient, who experienced an induced episode from the auditory stimuli, suddenly looked up at the ceiling with a fearful expression, started pointing about with one hand, and then proceeded to remove her electrodes with agitation. She later reported hearing someone tell her to tear away the electrodes, else she was going to suffocate because the electrodes were attached to the ceiling.

Less information exits concerning the phenomenology of sleep terrors, but some evidence suggests that if questioned immediately following an episode, patients may report indistinct recollections of immediate threats from which they were trying to escape. Precipitating imagery, ranging from a brief frightening image or thought to more elaborate dreamlike mentation, has been noted, particularly in adults.[7,16–18] Although some of this mental content may be related to postarousal states (eg, fear of dying associated with autonomic activation), there exist numerous examples of imagery occurring during prearousal events.[16]

These clinical observations should not be taken as indicating that patients' mental content directly precipitates somnambulism in and of itself. On the other hand, such reports raise important questions as to the role that phenomenological contents play in how somnambulistic episodes, and to a lesser extent sleep terrors, are experienced and unfold. In addition, these findings suggest that somnambulism should not be assumed to necessarily reflect automatic behaviors in the pure sense of the term and that morning recall of sleepwalking episodes may be greater than generally believed. Clinicians and researchers may thus gain valuable information by investigating these dimensions of experiences of people with parasomnia.

PSYCHOLOGICAL TESTING

The presence of somnambulism (with or without concomitant sleep terrors) in adulthood has often been viewed as a sign of major psychopathology.[19–21] In early childhood, the occurrence of somnambulism can be associated with separation anxiety.[22] In both children and adults, waking anxiety may also increase episode occurrence.[23–25] Psychopathology has been reported in subgroups of adolescents with sleep terrors and/or sleepwalk-ing.[26] One epidemiologic study found a higher prev-alence of psychopathology among adult patients with arousal disorders.[27] However, many adult patients with a history of NREM parasomnias do not present with a *DSM*-based[10] psychiatric disorder nor with highly disturbed personality traits.[7,28–30]

ASSESSMENT OF DAYTIME DYSFUNCTION

Although considerable research has focused on sleepwalkers' sleep electroencephalographic (EEG) results, virtually nothing is known about their daytime functioning. New lines of investigation provide evidence that adult sleepwalkers show dysfunctions during wakefulness. Using transcra-nial magnetic stimulation, one study[31] investigated motor cortex excitability during wakefulness in sleepwalkers and controls. Sleepwalkers showed significant hypoexcitability of some inhibitory circuits as revealed by reduced short-interval intracortical inhibition, cortical silent period duration, and short latency afferent inhibition. This innovative work suggests that transcranial magnetic stimulation, a technique widely used in clinical neurophysiology, may contribute to our understanding of the brain pathophysiology underlying NREM parasomnias.

Clinical experience with patients presenting with NREM parasomnias reveals that although these patients feel that they sleep well, many sleep-walkers complain of daytime somnolence. Similarly, one questionnaire-based investigation showed that half of the sleepwalkers questioned reported expe-riencing significant daytime somnolence.[14] The objective validly of these observations was recently supported by a study[32] showing that sleepwalkers have significantly lower mean sleep latencies on the multiple sleep latency test than age- and sex-matched control subjects. Moreover, 70% of the sleepwalkers and none of the controls had a mean latency less than 8 minutes, considered to be the threshold for clinical somnolence. Because the sleepwalkers investigated had a very low apnea-hypopnea index (0.70 ± 0.40), the daytime somno-lence is unlikely because of sleep-disordered breathing.

Excessive daytime sleepiness experienced by adult sleepwalkers may partially account for the intriguing findings from a large epidemiologic study[27] showing that people with sleepwalking were 5 times more likely to have an automobile accident during the past year than were people without parasomnias. Additional testing of daytime performance and vigilance in patients suffering from NREM arousal parasomnias is required to better understand the clinical and functional signif-icance of this daytime somnolence.

USE OF POLYSOMNOGRAPHY

When case presentations involve violent or injurious behaviors, excessive daytime sleepiness, or as-sociated medical or neurologic conditions, more extensive evaluations, including overnight poly-somnography with an expanded EEG montage, may be required. The polysomnogram can also be useful in ruling out other disorders (eg, nocturnal seizures, episodic nocturnal wandering, RBD) or in identifying primary sleep-related disorders (eg, sleep-disordered breathing, periodic limb move-ment disorder) that might underlie the parasomnia. In all cases, continuous audiovisual monitoring is essential to document behavioral manifestations and to correlate monitored events with polysomno-graphic characteristics.

Diagnosing NREM parasomnias directly with pol-ysomnography, however, is often difficult because episodes rarely occur in the sleep laboratory and the diagnosis cannot be ruled out based on a normal polysomnogram. Analyses of sleep architecture cycling among sleep stages reveal no significant or consistent differences between adult patients with somnambulism/sleep terror and control subjects, except for a greater number of arousals selectively out of SWS in those with parasomnia, even for nights without sleepwalking or sleep terror episodes (**Fig. 1**).[15,33–36] When compared with controls, adults and children with sleepwalking/sleep terrors show increases in the cyclic alter-nating pattern rate,[37–39] a measure of NREM instability. NREM sleep instability and arousal oscil-lation may represent a typical microstructural feature of NREM sleep of those with parasomnia. Other polysomnographic features including fre-quent presence of hypersynchronous delta waves and diminished slow wave activity (SWA) have been proposed as indirect evidence supporting the diagnosis, but these variables do not possess sufficient sensitivity and specificity.[40–42]

Experimental sleep deprivation can be used to trigger episodes of somnambulism in the sleep laboratory because these rarely occur spontane-ously in laboratory conditions. Two studies found that 24 and 38 hours of sleep deprivation signifi-cantly increased the frequency of somnambulistic events in sleepwalkers,[43,44] whereas one study did not find an increase in the number of episodes after 36 hours of sleep deprivation.[45] These incon-sistencies may be, in part, because of the limited number of patients investigated (7–10). A more recent investigation[46] of 40 sleepwalkers revealed that 25 hours of sleep deprivation was also effec-tive in increasing both the frequency and complexity of somnambulistic events recorded in the sleep laboratory. Combining data from all 40

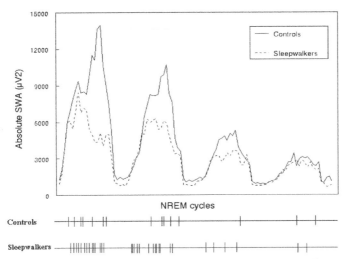

Fig. 1. Slow wave activity (SWA) over 4 consecutive NREM-REM cycles in 15 sleepwalkers and 15 healthy paired controls. Power is significantly reduced in the second half of the first NREM period. Awakenings from SWS are indicated on the 2 horizontal lines below the graph. (*From* Gaudreau H, Joncas S, Zadra A, et al. Dynamics of slow-wave activity during the NREM sleep of sleepwalkers and control subjects. Sleep 2000;23(6):755–60; with permission.)

patients shows that recovery sleep resulted in 1 or more episodes being recorded from 36 (90%) of the sleepwalkers. However, it should be noted that many of the recorded episodes were relatively simple manifestations such as playing with the bed sheets or the electrodes wires, turning and resting on one's hands while staring about with observable confusion, resting on one's knees, or trying to get out of bed. The fact that none of the control subjects investigated in these studies experienced nocturnal behavioral manifestations in the laboratory demonstrates that sleep deprivation alone does not lead to somnambulistic episodes but rather it increases the probability of somnambulistic behaviors in predisposed individuals.

There is also some support for the idea that forced arousals can be used to precipitate sleepwalking or sleep terrors in predisposed children or adults. Pilot studies of a few young sleepwalkers found that behavioral events could be induced by standing the child on his or her feet during SWS.[2,47–49] Two episodes were also triggered during SWS in 1 of the 4 children by calling the child's name.[48] In one study of patients with sleep terror, sounding a loud buzzer during SWS induced sleep terrors in 2 of 4 patients.[50]

The hypothesis combining factors that deepen sleep (eg, sleep deprivation) with those that fragment sleep (eg, environmental stimuli) increases the probability of sleepwalkers experiencing an episode was tested in a study of 10 adult sleepwalkers and 10 control subjects.[15] After a normal night of baseline recording in the sleep laboratory, night, participants

were presented with auditory stimuli during normal sleep or recovery sleep after 25 hours of sleep deprivation. Auditory stimuli (3 seconds of a pure sound at 1000 Hz) were delivered during different sleep stages according to a preestablished protocol in ascending intensities of 10 dB (40 dB–90 dB) with a minimal interval of 1 minute between 2 stimuli. Auditory stimuli were presented in the targeted sleep stage after at least 1 minute of stable EEG and electromyography until an EEG arousal, a behavioral episode, or a maximum of 6 auditory stimuli was reached. Stimulus presentations were performed with Neuroscan (Neurosoft Inc, Sterling, VA, USA), a software environment for custom stimulus presentation, and delivered with earphones inserted into subjects' ears.

The mean frequency of all somnambulistic events recorded across sleepwalkers' PSG assessments is presented in **Fig. 2**. Forced arousals during SWS were successful in experimentally inducing somnambulistic episodes in adult sleepwalkers, and, as predicted, sleep deprivation significantly increased the forced arousals' efficacy. Although no somnambulistic episodes were induced in controls, the presentation of auditory stimuli during daytime recovery sleep resulted in all 10 patients experiencing 1 or more induced episodes. The mean intensity of auditory stimuli that induced somnambulistic episodes during sleepwalkers' SWS was comparable to the mean intensity of auditory stimuli that induced full awakenings during both sleepwalkers' and controls' SWS (approximately 50 dB). This intensity is also

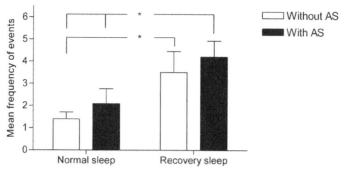

Fig. 2. Mean frequency (and standard error of the mean) of somnambulistic events recorded in sleepwalkers across sleep periods with and without auditory stimuli (AS). Differences are significant at a level of $P<.05$. Results show that the number of somnambulistic episodes significantly increases during recovery sleep with AS when compared with baseline and normal sleep with AS. Recovery sleep without AS also significantly increases the mean frequency of episodes when compared with baseline recordings. (*From* Pilon M, Montplaisir J, Zadra A, et al. Precipitating factors of somnambulism: impact of sleep deprivation and forced arousals. Neurology 2008;70(24):2284–90; with permission.)

consistent with studies having investigated auditory arousal thresholds in normal adults' SWS.[51,52] These findings thus suggest that sleepwalkers are neither more easily nor more difficult to awaken from SWS than are controls but rather that sleepwalkers suffer from an atypical and distinct arousal reaction.

Taken as a whole, these results support the hypothesis that via its homeostatic pressure for increased SWS, sleep deprivation facilitates the occurrence of sleepwalking in predisposed individuals and that this effect can be augmented by incorporating forced arousals during SWS.

BRAIN IMAGING

Over the past decade, positron emission tomography neuroimaging has provided an important tool to investigate subtle changes in cerebral blood flow (CBF) and metabolism throughout the human sleep-wake cycle.[53] For example, when compared with wakefulness or REM sleep,[54–58] NREM sleep is characterized by a global decrease in CBF and a regional CBF (rCBF) decrease in several regions, including the dorsal pons, mesencephalon, thalamus, basal ganglia, basal forebrain, anterior hypothalamus, prefrontal cortex, anterior cingulate cortex, and precuneus. However, few neuroimaging studies have been conducted in actual sleep-disordered patients, and its use as a diagnostic tool in such patients remains to be shown.

A single-case SPECT study was performed during a sleepwalking episode recorded from a 16-year-old adolescent boy with a history of somnambulism.[59] It showed an increase of 25% in rCBF in the posterior cingulate and anterior cerebellum compared with SWS without episodes. The

investigators suggest that variations in the motor and emotional manifestations of sleepwalking may be related to different activation patterns of the cingulate cortex because it modulates behavior in response to emotional processes. A decrease in rCBF in frontoparietal associative cortices was also noted in comparison with the wakefulness pattern of normal subjects. The EEG recorded during the episode showed diffuse high-voltage rhythmic delta activity. These pilot findings support the view of sleepwalking, a dissociated state consisting of motor arousal and persisting mind sleep. Although this line of neuroimaging research may help us understand the basis for the lack of self-awareness, judgment, and confusion that typifies many somnambulistic episodes, its ease of use and value in a clinical assessment or diagnosis of NREM parasomnias remains to be demonstrated.

DIFFERENTIAL DIAGNOSIS

Disorders of arousal need to be distinguished from RBD, nightmare disorder, complex partial seizures, and nocturnal panic attacks. RBD is characterized by intermittent loss of REM sleep atonia and by the appearance of elaborate motor activity associated with dream mentation during REM sleep. Patients usually have a vivid recall of the dreams that appear to correlate with observed behaviors. RBD can be also be distinguished from NREM parasomnias by its usual occurrence during the second half of the night and by the absence of mental confusion on awakening. However, some patients may have behavioral manifestations during both REM and NREM sleep, with RBD occurring in combination with a disorder of arousal. This condition is known as parasomnia overlap disorder.[29]

Nightmares are vivid and disturbing mental experiences that generally occur during REM sleep and often result in awakening.[1] They can be distinguished from sleep terrors by their usual occurrence during the second half of the night, when REM is most prominent, and by the recall of detailed dream content. The degree of automatic activation (eg, palpitations and dyspnea) is much greater during sleep terrors, and there is an absence of mental confusion on awakening from a nightmare as opposed to a sleep terror. Actual screaming or other intense vocalizations that can characterize sleep terrors are rare during nightmares.

Disorders of arousal and complex partial epileptic seizures share several clinical similarities, including sudden onset, unresponsiveness, and retrograde amnesia. In addition, these conditions are all sensitive to factors that deepen sleep, such as sleep deprivation. Nocturnal frontal lobe epilepsy can be particularly difficult to differentiate from NREM parasomnias, especially in children.[60,61] Complex partial seizures usually involve repetitive stereotypic behaviors, and patients rarely return to bed. Epileptic seizures may occur in any sleep stages throughout the sleep period. Similar seizure activity may occur during daytime wakefulness. Sleep terrors and seizures may coexist in the same person.

Approximately 50% of all patients with panic disorder have nocturnal panic attacks that are characterized by intense fear or discomfort accompanied by cognitive and physical symptoms of arousal.[10] These attacks are comparable with panic attacks experienced in the daytime, and they may sometimes be clinically similar to sleep terrors. Nocturnal panic attacks usually occur in late stage 2 or early stage 3 sleep, and, unlike many sleep terrors, patients do not become physically agitated or aggressive during the panic attack.[62] Immediately after a nocturnal panic attack, patients are oriented, can vividly recall their attack, and usually have difficulty returning to sleep (ie, suffer from insomnia); these features differ from those observed in patients with sleep terrors.

Sleep Disorders

In both children and adults, sleepwalking and sleep terrors can be secondary to sleep respiratory events, including obstructive sleep apnea and upper airway resistance syndrome, or other sleep disorders.[27,30,63–65] Treatment of the precipitating sleep disorder (eg, continuous positive airway pressure for sleep-disordered breathing) can result in a disappearance of the disorder of arousal.[30,64]

However, some studies find that that a majority of adult sleepwalkers do not suffer from comorbid sleep disorders.[46]

NREM Parasomnias Associated with Medical Conditions

Rarely, NREM parasomnias may develop as a result of medical or neurologic conditions. One study[66] reported 6 cases of adult-onset (de novo) sleepwalking in patients with Parkinson disease. De novo sleep terrors have been reported in association with right thalamic lesion[67] and brainstem lesion.[68] De novo somnambulism has also been described in patients presenting with thyrotoxicosis caused by diffuse toxic goiter or Graves disease.[69,70] Disorders of arousal can also be triggered by medication, including sedatives/hypnotics, neuroleptics, lithium, minor tranquilizers, stimulants, and antihistamines.

It should also be noted that hormonal factors may influence the frequency with which women experience NREM arousal disorders because these disorders can emerge premenstrually[71] or decrease during pregnancy, particularly in primiparas.[72]

CLINICAL VARIANTS: SLEEP-RELATED EATING DISORDER AND SLEEP-RELATED ABNORMAL SEXUAL BEHAVIORS

The behaviors manifested during an arousal disorder can be relatively distinct and specialized. Two variants of NREM parasomnias involve sleep-related eating disorder (SRED) and sleep-related abnormal sexual behaviors (SRASBs).

According to the *International Classification of Sleep Disorders*,[1] SRED, classified under the "Other Parasomnia" section, consists of recurrent episodes of involuntary eating and drinking during arousal from sleep with problematic consequences. Episodes typically occur during partial arousals from sleep during the first third of the night with varying degrees of awareness and impaired recall.[73–75] Polysomnographic studies have associated SRED with a variety of underlying sleep disorders, the most frequent of which is sleepwalking. SRED can also be associated with restless leg syndrome, periodic limb movements of sleep, obstructive sleep apnea, and circadian rhythm disorders.[73,74] SRED has also been reported in association with medications such as zolpidem or triazolam.

SRASBs, also known as sexsomnia or sleep sex, consist of inappropriate sexual activities occurring without conscious awareness during sleep.[76,77] SRASBs can range from sexual vocalizations or sexualized bodily movements to violent masturbation or sexual assaults and have been reported as being markedly different from behaviors normally initiated during the patient's waking state.[78,79] According to the *ICSD-II*,[1] SRASB is classified in the "Disorders of Arousal" section as a clinical subtype of confusional arousal. Disorders of arousal, and sleepwalking in particular, are the most frequent sleep disorders associated with SRASB, although it could also occur in association with RBD or NREM complex partial seizures.[78,80] As detailed elsewhere (Schenck and colleagues, 2007), a wide range of sleep-related disorders may be associated with SRASB.

SUMMARY

Despite numerous clinical and empirical investigations, the exact mechanisms that give rise to NREM parasomnias remain unclear. A strong genetic component has been well documented and patients with NREM arousal parasomnias also experience difficulties maintaining stable and consolidated NREM sleep. Diagnostic methods remain largely confined to clinical interviews and presenting history. Assessment of phenomenological dimensions associated with somnambulism and sleep terrors indicates that sleep mentation can play an important role in the subjective experience of these 2 parasomnias. The use of sleep deprivation (with or without experimentally induced forced arousals) can help capture actual episodes in the sleep laboratory, but no validated protocol exists to directly confirm the diagnosis. The limited data collected with neuroimaging and transcranial magnetic stimulation in relation to NREM parasomnias suggest that, although methodologically challenging, these investigative tools may pave the way toward a better understanding of disorders of arousal.

REFERENCES

1. American Academy of Sleep Medicine. ICSD-2: the international classification of sleep disorders: diagnostic and coding manual. 2nd edition. Westchester (IL): American Academy of Sleep Medicine; 2005.
2. Broughton RJ. Sleep disorders: disorders of arousal? Science 1968;159(3819):1070–8.
3. Hublin C, Kaprio J, Partinen M, et al. Parasomnias: co-occurrence and genetics. Psychiatr Genet 2001;11(2):65–70.
4. Hublin C, Kaprio J. Genetic aspects and genetic epidemiology of parasomnias. Sleep Med Rev 2003;7(5):413–21.
5. Lecendreux M, Bassetti C, Dauvilliers Y, et al. HLA and genetic susceptibility to sleepwalking. Mol Psychiatry 2003;8(1):114–7.
6. Licis A, Desruisseau D, Yamada K, et al. Novel genetic findings in an extended family pedigree with sleepwalking. Neurology 2011;76:49–52.
7. Schenck CH, Milner DM, Hurwitz TD, et al. A polysomnographic and clinical report on sleep-related injury in 100 adult patients. Am J Psychiatry 1989;146(9):1166–73.
8. Siclarim F, Khatami R, Urbanoik F, et al. Violence in sleep. Brain 2010;133:3494–509.
9. Ohayon MM, Schenck CH. Violent behavior during sleep: prevalence, comorbidity and consequences. Sleep Med 2010;11:941–6.
10. APA. Diagnostic and statistical manual of mental disorders: DSM-IV. 4th edition. Washington, DC: American Psychiatric Association; 1994.
11. Bornemann MC, Mahowald MW. Sleep forensics. In: Kryger M, Roth T, Dement WC, editors. Principles and practice of sleep medicine. 5th edition. St Louis (MO): Elsevier; 2011. p. 725–33.
12. Vignatelli L, Bisulli F, Zaniboni A, et al. Interobserver reliability of ICSD-R minimal diagnostic criteria for the parasomnias. J Neurol 2005;252(6):712–7.
13. Zadra A, Pilon M, Montplaisir J. Phenomenological experiences in adult sleepwalkers. Towards a Science of Consciousness, Research Abstracts 2008;126.
14. Oudiette D, Leu S, Pottier M, et al. Dreamlike mentations during sleepwalking and sleep terrors in adults. Sleep 2009;32(12):1621–7.
15. Pilon M, Montplaisir J, Zadra A, et al. Precipitating factors of somnambulism: impact of sleep deprivation and forced arousals. Neurology 2008;70(24):2284–90.
16. Fisher C, Kahn E, Edwards A, et al. A psychophysiological study of nightmares and night terrors: III. Mental content and recall of stage 4 night terrors. J Nerv Ment Dis 1974;158(3):174–88.
17. Kahn E, Fisher C, Edwards A. Night terrors and anxiety dreams. In: Ellman SJ, Antrobus JS, editors. The mind in sleep: psychology and psychophysiology. 2nd edition. New York: Wiley Interscience: John Wiley & Sons; 1991. p. 437–47.
18. Pressman MR. Disorders of arousal from sleep and violent behavior: the role of physical contact and proximity. Sleep 2007;30(8):1039–47.
19. Soldatos CR, Vela-Bueno A, Bixler EO, et al. Sleepwalking and night terrors in adulthood clinical EEG findings. Clin Electroencephalogr 1980;11(3):136–9.
20. Pai MN. Sleep-walking and sleep activities. J Ment Sci 1946;92:756–65.
21. Kales A, Soldatos CR, Caldwell AB, et al. Somnambulism. Clinical characteristics and personality patterns. Arch Gen Psychiatry 1980;37(12):1406–10.
22. Petit D, Touchette E, Tremblay RE, et al. Dyssomnias and parasomnias in early childhood. Pediatrics 2007;119(5):e1016–25.
23. Rosen G, Mahowald MW, Ferber R. Sleepwalking, confusional arousals, and sleep terrors in the child. In: Ferber R, Kryger M, editors. Principles and

practice of sleep medicine in the child. Philadelphia: WB Saunders Company; 1995. p. 99–106.

24. Cirignotta F, Zucconi M, Mondini S, et al. Enuresis, sleepwalking, and nightmares: an epidemiological survey in the republic of San Marino. In: Guilleminault C, Lugaresi E, editors. Sleep/wake disorder: natural history, epidemiology, and long-term evolution. New York: Raven Press; 1983. p. 237–41.

25. Crisp AH, Matthews BM, Oakey M, et al. Sleepwalking, night terrors, and consciousness. BMJ 1990; 300(6721):360–2.

26. Gau SF, Soong WT. Psychiatric comorbidity of adolescents with sleep terrors or sleepwalking: a case-control study. Aust N Z J Psychiatry 1999; 33(5):734–9.

27. Ohayon MM, Guilleminault C, Priest RG. Night terrors, sleepwalking, and confusional arousals in the general population: their frequency and relationship to other sleep and mental disorders. J Clin Psychiatry 1999;60(4):268–76 [quiz: 277].

28. Mahowald MW, Schenck CH. Dissociated states of wakefulness and sleep. In: Lydic R, Baghdoyan HA, editors. Handbook of behavioural state control: cellular and molecular mechanisms. New York: CRC Press; 1999. p. 143–58.

29. Schenck CH, Boyd JL, Mahowald MW. A parasomnia overlap disorder involving sleepwalking, sleep terrors, and REM sleep behavior disorder in 33 polysomnographically confirmed cases. Sleep 1997; 20(11):972–81.

30. Guilleminault C, Kirisoglu C, Bao G, et al. Adult chronic sleepwalking and its treatment based on polysomnography. Brain 2005;128(Pt 5):1062–9.

31. Oliviero A, Della Marca G, Tonali PA, et al. Functional involvement of cerebral cortex in adult sleepwalking. J Neurol 2007;254(8):1066–72.

32. Montplaisir J, Petit D, Pilon M, et al. Does sleepwalking impair daytime vigilance? J Clin Sleep Med 2011;7:219.

33. Blatt I, Peled R, Gadoth N, et al. The value of sleep recording in evaluating somnambulism in young adults. Electroencephalogr Clin Neurophysiol 1991; 78(6):407–12.

34. Espa F, Ondze B, Deglise P, et al. Sleep architecture, slow wave activity, and sleep spindles in adult patients with sleepwalking and sleep terrors. Clin Neurophysiol 2000;111(5):929–39.

35. Halasz P, Ujszaszi J, Gadoros J. Are microarousals preceded by electroencephalographic slow wave synchronization precursors of confusional awakenings? Sleep 1985;8(3):231–8.

36. Gaudreau H, Joncas S, Zadra A, et al. Dynamics of slow-wave activity during the NREM sleep of sleepwalkers and control subjects. Sleep 2000;23(6):755–60.

37. Zucconi M, Oldani A, Ferini-Strambi L, et al. Arousal fluctuations in non-rapid eye movement parasomnias: the role of cyclic alternating pattern as

a measure of sleep instability. J Clin Neurophysiol 1995;12(2):147–54.

38. Guilleminault C, Lee JH, Chan A, et al. Non-REM sleep instability in recurrent sleepwalking in prepubertal children. Sleep Med 2005;6:515–21.

39. Bruni O, Ferri R, Novelli L, et al. NREM sleep instability in children with sleep terrors: the role of slow wave activity interruptions. Clin Neurophysiol 2008; 119(5):985–92.

40. Pressman MR. Factors that predispose, prime and precipitate NREM parasomnias in adults: clinical and forensic implications. Sleep Med Rev 2007; 11(1):5–30.

41. Pilon M, Zadra A, Joncas S, et al. Hypersynchronous delta waves and somnambulism: brain topography and effect of sleep deprivation. Sleep 2006;29:77–84.

42. Pressman MR. Hypersynchronous delta sleep EEG activity and sudden arousals from slow-wave sleep in adults without a history of parasomnias: clinical and forensic implications. Sleep 2004;27(4):706–10.

43. Joncas S, Zadra A, Paquet J, et al. The value of sleep deprivation as a diagnostic tool in adult sleepwalkers. Neurology 2002;58(6):936–40.

44. Mayer G, Neissner V, Schwarzmayr P, et al. Sleep deprivation in somnambulism. Effect of arousal, deep sleep and sleep stage changes. Nervenarzt 1998;69(6):495–501 [in German].

45. Guilleminault C, Leger D, Philip P, et al. Nocturnal wandering and violence: review of a sleep clinic population. J Forensic Sci 1998;43(1):158–63.

46. Zadra A, Pilon M, Montplaisir J, et al. Polysomnographic diagnosis of sleepwalking: effects of sleep deprivation. Ann Neurol 2008;63(4):513–9.

47. Gastaut H, Broughton RJ. A clinical and polygraphic study of episodic phenomena during sleep. Recent Adv Biol Psychiatry 1965;7:197–223.

48. Kales A, Jacobson A, Paulson MJ, et al. Somnambulism: psychophysiological correlates. I. All-night EEG studies. Arch Gen Psychiatry 1966;14(6):586–94.

49. Jacobson A, Kales A. Somnambulism: all-night EEG and related studies. Res Publ Assoc Res Nerv Ment Dis 1967;45:424–55.

50. Fisher C, Kahn E, Edwards A, et al. A psychophysiological study of nightmares and night terrors. I. Physiological aspects of the stage 4 night terror. J Nerv Ment Dis 1973;157(2):75–98.

51. Williams HL, Hammack JT, Caly RL, et al. Responses to auditory stimulation, sleep loss and the EEG stages of sleep. Electroencephalogr Clin Neurophysiol 1964;16:269–79.

52. Rosa RR, Bonnet MH. Sleep stages, auditory arousal threshold, and body temperature as predictors of behavior upon awakening. Int J Neurosci 1985;27(1–2):73–83.

53. Dang-Vu TT, Desseilles M, Petit D, et al. Neuroimaging in sleep medicine. Sleep Med 2007;8(4): 349–72.

54. Maquet P, Degueldre C, Delfiore G, et al. Functional neuroanatomy of human slow wave sleep. J Neurosci 1997;17(8):2807–12.

55. Maquet P. Functional neuroimaging of normal human sleep by positron emission tomography. J Sleep Res 2000;9(3):207–31.

56. Braun AR, Balkin TJ, Wesenten NJ, et al. Regional cerebral blood flow throughout the sleep-wake cycle. An H2(15)O PET study. Brain 1997;120(Pt 7): 1173–97.

57. Kajimura N, Uchiyama M, Takayama Y, et al. Activity of midbrain reticular formation and neocortex during the progression of human non-rapid eye movement sleep. J Neurosci 1999;19(22):10065–73.

58. Andersson JL, Onoe H, Hetta J, et al. Brain networks affected by synchronized sleep visualized by positron emission tomography. J Cereb Blood Flow Metab 1998;18(7):701–15.

59. Bassetti C, Vella S, Donati F, et al. SPECT during sleepwalking. Lancet 2000;356(9228):484–5.

60. Zucconi M, Ferini-Strambi L. NREM parasomnias: arousal disorders and differentiation from nocturnal frontal lobe epilepsy. Clin Neurophysiol 2000; 111(Suppl 2):S129–35.

61. Derry CP, Harvey AS, Walker MC, et al. NREM arousal parasomnias and their distinction from nocturnal frontal lobe epilepsy: a video EEG analysis. Sleep 2009;32(12):1637–44.

62. Craske MG, Tsao JC. Assessment and treatment of nocturnal panic attacks. Sleep Med Rev 2005;9(3): 173–84.

63. Espa F, Dauvilliers Y, Ondze B, et al. Arousal reactions in sleepwalking and night terrors in adults: the role of respiratory events. Sleep 2002;25(8): 871–5.

64. Guilleminault C, Palombini L, Pelayo R, et al. Sleepwalking and sleep terrors in prepubertal children: what triggers them? Pediatrics 2003;111(1):e17–25.

65. Goodwin J, Kaemingh K, Fregosi R, et al. Parasomnias and sleep disordered breathing in Caucasian and Hispanic children—the Tucson children's assessment of sleep apnea study. BMC Med 2004; 2:14.

66. Poryazova R, Waldvogel D, Bassetti CL, et al. Sleepwalking in patients with Parkinson disease. Arch Neurol 2007;64(10):1524–7.

67. Di Gennaro G, Autret A, Mascia A, et al. Night terrors associated with thalamic lesion. Clin Neurophysiol 2004;115(11):2489–92.

68. Mendez MF. Pavor nocturnus from a brainstem glioma. J Neurol Neurosurg Psychiatry 1992;55(9):860.

69. Ajlouni KM, Ahmad AT, Al-Zahiri MM, et al. Sleepwalking associated with hyperthyroidism. Endocr Pract 2005;11(1):5–10.

70. Ajlouni K, Daradkeh TK, Ajlouni H, et al. De novo sleepwalking associated with hyperthyroidism. Sleep Hypn 2001;3(3):112–6.

71. Schenck CH, Mahowald MW. Two cases of premenstrual sleep terrors and injurious sleep-walking. J Psychosom Obstet Gynaecol 1995;16(2):79–84.

72. Hedman C, Pohjasvaara T, Tolonen U, et al. Parasomnias decline during pregnancy. Acta Neurol Scand 2002;105(3):209–14.

73. Schenck C, Hurwitz T, O'Connor K, et al. Additional categories of sleep-related eating disorders and the current status of treatment. Sleep 1993;16(5):457–66.

74. Winkelman JW. Clinical and polysomnographic features of sleep-related eating disorder. J Clin Psychiatry 1998;59(1):14–9.

75. Howell MJ, Schenck C, Crow SJ. A review of nighttime eating disorders. Sleep Med Rev 2009;13:23–34.

76. Mahowald MW, Schenck CH, Cramer Bornemann MA. Sleep-related violence. Curr Neurol Neurosci Rep 2005;5(2):153–8.

77. Andersen ML, Poyares D, Alves RS, et al. Sexsomnia: abnormal sexual behavior during sleep. Brain Res 2007;56(2):271–82.

78. Guilleminault C, Moscovitch A, Yuen K, et al. Atypical sexual behavior during sleep. Psychosom Med 2002;64(2):328–36.

79. Shapiro CM, Trajanovic NN, Fedoroff J. Sexsomnia: a new parasomnia? Can J Psychiatry 2003;48(5):311–7.

80. Schenck CH, Arnulf I, Mahowald MW. Sleep and sex: what can go wrong? A review of the literature on sleep related disorders and abnormal sexual behaviors and experiences. Sleep 2007;30(6):683–702.

REM Sleep Behavior Disorder

Naoko Tachibana, MD, PhD[a,b,]*

KEYWORDS

- Parasomnia • REM sleep behavior disorder
- Polysomnography • REM sleep without atonia
- Synucleinopathy

Rapid eye movement (REM) sleep behavior disorder (RBD) is a REM sleep-related parasomnia, characterized by dream-enacted behaviors ranging from simple vocalizations or mumbling sleep talk to full-blown violent behaviors leading to injuries of the patient and/or the bed partner. The polysomnographic hallmark of RBD is the intermittent or sustained loss of the skeletal muscle atonia of REM sleep (REM sleep without atonia [RWA]), and this finding is mandatory in the diagnostic criteria (requiring polysomnographic [PSG] monitoring) in the International Classification of Sleep Disorders-2 (ICSD-2) (**Box 1**).[1] RBD has attracted the attention of sleep researchers and sleep medicine clinicians for three reasons. First, this disorder provides insight about the mechanism of REM sleep generation in humans. Second, it affects the quality of life of the patients as well as their bed partners with social embarrassment, psychological conflict, and the possibility of injuries. Third, most RBD is associated with various neurologic disorders, especially with neurodegenerative diseases known as synucleinopathy, including Parkinson disease (PD), dementia with Lewy bodies (LBD), and multiple system atrophy (MSA).[2,3] This last aspect of RBD has also become a matter of interest for neurologists or movement disorder specialists, because RBD is often an antecedent of the onset (motor and/or cognitive manifestation) of synucleinopathy. This suggests future hope of neuroprotective treatment in some RBD patients who are considered in early stages of these neurodegenerative diseases.

EPIDEMIOLOGY AND DEMOGRAPHICS

There have been only two published epidemiologic studies with relevance to RBD in the general population.[4,5] One study was based on telephone interviews, in the United Kingdom, of 4972 individuals aged 15 to 100 years. The other study was done with a two-stage design using a sleep-related injury question for the first step. The suspected subjects were then invited to undergo polysomnographic testing. These studies estimated that RBD occurred in 0.5% or 0.38% of patients, respectively. In clinical settings, there were 67 RBD patients (0.6%) confirmed by polysomnography out of 10,745 consecutive patients during 8 years. These patients came to an independent sleep center in a general hospital in Japan where direct self-referral was the norm.[6] Studies of large case series indicated that there was a higher prevalence in older age, usually over age 60 years, with male predominance.[6–9] However, the frequency is much higher in certain neurodegenerative diseases, especially PD, LBD, and MSA.[2,3,10]

CLINICAL FEATURES

RBD is characterized by complex and elaborate motor activity often associated with agitated and violent dream mentation. The content of the dream usually consists of being attacked, threatened, or chased by unfamiliar people or villains; dangerous animals such as dogs, snakes, tigers, and lions; or imaginative monsters. However, the nonemotional

The author has nothing to disclose.
a Center for Sleep-related Disorders, Kansai Electric Power Hospital, 2-1-7 Fukushima, Fukushima, Osaka 553-0003, Japan
b Tokushima University Graduate School of Medicine, 3-18-15 Kuramoto, Tokushima 770-8503, Japan
* Center for Sleep-related Disorders, Kansai Electric Power Hospital, 2-1-7 Fukushima, Fukushima, Osaka 553-0003, Japan.
E-mail address: nanaosaka@aol.com

Sleep Med Clin 6 (2011) 459–468
doi:10.1016/j.jsmc.2011.08.009

Box 1
Diagnostic criteria of REM sleep behavior disorder

1. Presence of REM sleep without atonia on PSG

2. At least one of the following:

   a. Sleep-related, injurious, potentially injurious, or disruptive behaviors by history (ie, dream-enactment behavior)

   b. Abnormal REM sleep behavior documented during polysomnographic monitoring

3. Absence of EEG epileptiform activity during REM sleep unless RBD can be clearly distinguished from any concurrent REM sleep-related seizure disorder

4. The sleep disorder is cannot be better explained by another sleep disorder, medical or neurologic disorder, mental disorder, medication use, or substance use disorder.

---

or neutral nature of dream content does not exclude the diagnosis. Many patients are able to recall and describe the dream content when being awakened during or immediately after the behaviors, but some only remember that they had a dream with very vague content in the morning.

Patients with RBD demonstrate a wide spectrum of abnormal dream-enacted behaviors ranging from simple verbalization to complex motor phenomena.[7–9] Noncomplex behaviors can also occur in RBD patients.[11] When the behavior is relatively subtle in nature such as mumbling and small jerky movements of the limbs, it does not usually bringing the patient to the attention of a sleep physician. However, when RBD consists of more agitated and harmful behaviors such as yelling, shouting, screaming, punching, kicking, jumping, and running out of the bed that correlate with the reported aggressive dream imaginary experience, the bed partner should seek consultation, especially when the injury is related to episodes. The repertoire of behaviors and dream contents do not much differ between patients with apparent idiopathic RBD (iRBD) and those with MSA or PD.[12]

During these events, the eyes are usually closed because the patient is attending to the dream content instead of to the bedside environment. Therefore, if the bed partner tried to stop the behaviors of the patient by physical contact, this could trigger more intense violence because the patient would react against this attempt to abort

the event, considering the bed partner a threatening intruder into the dream. RBD patients rarely leave the bedroom, but violent episodes sometimes have resulted in forensic issues.[13]

So long as the normal sleep structure is preserved (ie, cyclic appearance of non-REM [NREM] and REM sleep), RBD events tend to occur in the latter third of the sleep period. However, this rule is not always the case with RBD patients with narcolepsy, severe sleep apnea syndrome, or in advanced stage of neurodegenerative diseases.

DIAGNOSTIC CRITERIA AND POLYSOMNOGRAPHIC FEATURES

RBD was added to the International Classification of Sleep Disorders (ICSD) in 1990 as a parasomnia, and in the present ICSD-2 is described in detail.[1] In ICSD-2, documentation of RWA by PSG is required. RWA is empirically defined as excessive amounts of sustained or intermittent elevation of submental electromyogram (EMG) tone or excessive phasic submental EMG twitching with the other features of REM sleep; that is, desynchronized EEG and rapid eye movements (**Fig. 1**). According to the new "American Academy of Sleep Medicine Manual for the Scoring of Sleep and Related Events,"[14] RWA can be scored when there is (1) sustained muscle activity in REM sleep with 50% of one epoch having increased chin EMG amplitude and/or (2) excessive transient muscle activity present in five or more mini-epochs (a conventional epoch of 30 seconds is divided into ten 3-second mini-epochs and transient muscle activity is defined as EMG activity lasting at least 0.5 seconds).

However, there is no standardized rule for which muscles should be used for analysis and, on some occasions, RBD patients demonstrate behaviors without chin muscle atonia, but with phasic muscle twitching of the limbs (**Fig. 2**). One study done by the Sleep-Innsbruck-Barcelona (SINBAR) group demonstrated that simultaneous recording of the mentalis, flexor digitorum superficialis, and extensor digitorum brevis muscles detected the highest rate of phasic EMG activity during REM sleep in subjects with RBD.[15]

DIFFERENTIAL DIAGNOSIS

Differential diagnosis is summarized in **Box 2**. Non-REM parasomnias (ie, sleep walking, night terrors, confusional arousals) are also characterized with complex behaviors during sleep. However, they tend to occur in the first third of the night and are usually not associated with elaborate dream

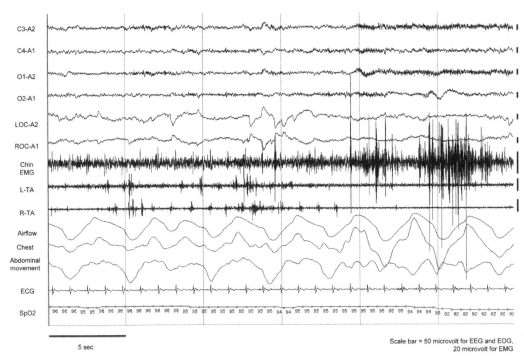

Fig. 1. A PSG strip scored as stage RWA recorded in an idiopathic RBD patient. The recording shows sustained elevation of submental EMG. LOC, outer canthus of the left eye; ROC, outer canthus of the right eye; TA, tibialis anterior.

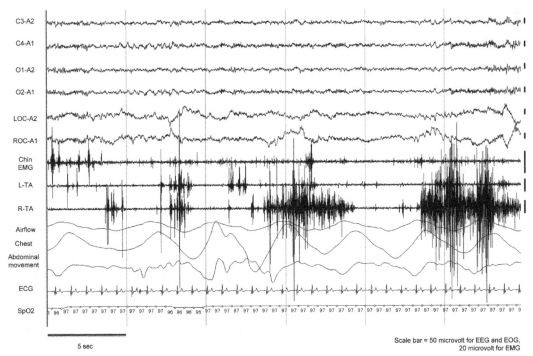

Fig. 2. A PSG strip from the patient of **Fig. 1** when he presented some jerky movements of the limbs. Chin EMG activity is suppressed with minimal phasic contamination, but there is excessive limb muscle twitching. LOC, outer canthus of the left eye; ROC, outer canthus of the right eye; TA, tibialis anterior.

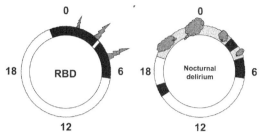

Fig. 3. A 24-hour clock for comparing nocturnal delirium with RBD. Nocturnal events of RBD are of short duration, occurring intermittently after sleeping some hours in accordance with preserved cycle of REM sleep. In nocturnal delirium, the events are continuous and the difference between sleep and wakefulness is ambiguous and often accompanied by disturbed sleep–wake rhythm.

enactment. Patients with non-REM sleep parasomnias look confused with eyes open during the behaviors and have no recall. Although there have been few reports, "parasomnia overlap disorder," which presents with combined features of sleepwalking, sleep terrors, and RBD, is also in the list of differential diagnosis.[16]

Vigorous body movements associated with vocalization may be noticed when patients with obstructive sleep apnea (OSA) resume breathing at the termination of respiratory events. Severe OSA patients may demonstrate dream-enacting behaviors and unpleasant dreams suggesting the diagnosis of RBD.[17] RBD and OSA can be coexistent and, in such a case, the possibility of RBD should be reevaluated after OSA has been treated.

Nocturnal epilepsy, especially nocturnal fontal lobe epilepsy (NFLE), often occurs exclusively during sleep, but NFLE is usually stereotypical and a lack of association with dream contents is the rule. The phenomenology of NFLE has been extensively described by the Bologna group as three types of events (paroxysmal arousals, nocturnal paroxysmal dystonia, and episodic nocturnal wanderings) and video- electroencephalogram [EEG]-PSG recording is useful if this diagnosis is suspected.[18] Alternatively, RBD may coexist in the elderly with epilepsy.[19,20] Nocturnal delirium is usually more continuous and the patients are disoriented and disconnected from the environment, whereas RBD episodes are intermittently observed during sleep and the patients have generally good orientation immediately after they are aroused (**Fig. 3**). However, this rule is not always the case—RBD patients may also suffer significant cognitive impairment and disturbed sleep–wake schedule (ie, advanced stage of LBD). Sleep-related dissociated disorders may present with various purposeful behaviors, during which episodes the patients show awake EEG with alpha rhythm. In any case, to make a correct diagnosis, a PSG with simultaneous video recording is mandatory.

PATHOPHYSIOLOGY

It is difficult to discuss the pathophysiology of RBD because the precise anatomic substrate and biochemical mechanisms of REM sleep itself are still in the process of clarification. The present hypothesized pathophysiology of RBD in humans is derived from a combination of widely investigated animal models in cats and rats[21–24] as well as recent physiologic and pathologic findings of neurodegenerative diseases with which RBD is frequently associated. Comprehensive reviews of elucidating RBD pathophysiology and related controversies from the viewpoint of RBD-neurodegenerative disease association can be found elsewhere.[2,3,25]

The principal hypothesized pathophysiology of RBD is that the pontine tegmentum and medial medulla are critical areas for muscle atonia, not only for mediating muscle atonia via active inhibition of spinal motor neurons, but also for suppressing locomotor activity. Therefore, when the involved neurons and/or pathways are anatomically or neurochemically disturbed, various motor phenomena are released during REM sleep.[26–31] This hypothesis is based on the assumption that the involved neural substrates in humans are similar to the animal models and that there have been accumulated reports about human RBD cases caused by a structural bilateral or unilateral focal lesions confined to the brainstem.[32–38] However, there have been no symptomatic studies that investigated the clinical sleep features, including nocturnal events and dreams and polysomnographic characteristics of REM sleep in patients with distinct lesions in the brainstem, such as cases of stroke or multiple sclerosis.

In the early days of RBD discovery, it was already known that half of RBD cases were associated with neurologic disorders.[7] Sleep investigators tried to attribute this to anatomic or functional disruptions of the substrates of REM-related muscle atonia. In 1996, Schenck and colleagues[39] presented the first prospective study to show that 38% of apparent idiopathic RBD patients had developed parkinsonian disorders with a mean interval of 12.7 years. Later, confirming studies established that a substantial number of iRBD patients eventually developed specific neurodegenerative diseases pathologically known as synucleinopathy (PD, LBD, and MSA).[2,40–42] In addition, more extensive studies have been done to demonstrate that polysomnographically proven RBD and/or RWA coexisted in PD (46%–58%),[43–46] and MSA (90.5%–100%).[12,47,48] The frequency of RBD and/or RWA documented by PSG in patients with LBD has not been well established, probably owing to the difficulty performing PSGs on consecutive patients with dementia. However, a series of studies by the Mayo group has demonstrated that RBD is one of the most important features to differentiate LBD from Alzheimer disease in patients with dementia.[49–53]

From these lines of evidence, iRBD, even if it may not present in all patients, is considered one of the prodromal symptoms of synucleinopathy and this notion has been strongly backed up by Braak's hypothesis.[54] Although this hypothesis does not mention that distinct lesions could result in REM sleep-related atonia, pathologic changes of caudal-rostral topographic sequence for PD can explain some cases in which RBD precedes parkinsonism and the lesions in the brainstem are compatible with animal studies.[2,25]

Alternately, neurologic disorders with no lesions in the brainstem have also been reported to coexist with RBD. Examples of these diseases are narcolepsy,[55–57] familial fatal insomnia,[58,59] and limbic encephalitis including Morvan chorea.[59–61] Because the nature and sites of the pathology of these diseases are different, it may not be possible to explain their pathophysiology by the experimental animal studies alone. However, all the involved anatomic structures of these diseases (narcolepsy, posterior hypothalamus; familial fatal insomnia, anterior thalamus; limbic encephalitis, limbic system) have neuronal projections to the brain stem nuclei. This suggests anatomic and/or functional dysregulation due to the primary pathology may result in RBD.

Finally, there have been many reports in the literature documenting pharmacologically induced RBD or RWA.[62–64] The secondary cause that has been most frequently reported is antidepressant therapy, but the pathophysiological mechanism is not clear. Most of these reports were anecdotal and the effect of discontinuation of antidepressants on RBD or RWA varied or was not well described.[64]

MANAGEMENT OF RBD

Whether and how we should treat a particular RBD patient depends on the severity of aggressive behavior, the degree of unpleasantness of the dreams, and the disturbed sleep quality of the bed partner. Treatment is targeted at preventing injuries and destruction of property, decreasing frequency, neutralizing contents of the dreams, and ensuring good quality of sleep for both the patient and bed partner.

Nonpharmacologic Intervention

Before commencing any treatment, an explanation of the nature of RBD to the patient is very important, assuring the patient that they are neither insane nor experiencing personality changes. Once the patient and bed partner understand that the behaviors are related to dreaming sleep, realistic treatment goals are easier to be determined. Even if the behaviors so far have not been violent (ie, only sleep talk and jerky movements of the limbs), patients must be warned about the potential for injury. Safety measures are necessary for all the patients who experienced injuries or presented potentially harmful behaviors.

Safety measures in the sleeping environment include sleeping in separate beds, no other furniture than beds in the bedroom, and placing a mattress on the floor alongside the bed. However, pharmacologic treatment should be started if a patient has already devised and tried a device such as special belts to tie himself or herself down to the bed. Clearly this type of improvement in environmental safety is strongly culturally bound. For example, in Japan, almost all couples have opted to sleep in separate bedrooms and on the futon mattress on the floor (personal observation).

Pharmacologic Treatment

Although no prospective placebo-controlled trials have been performed for any drugs for RBD other than one recent study,[65] two principal drugs have been widely used. One is clonazepam and the other melatonin.[66,67]

Open-label studies of clonazepam (0.25 mg–1 mg at bedtime) have suggested that it is effective in approximately 90% of the patients with little evidence of tolerance or abuse, regardless if idiopathic or symptomatic.[8,68,69] Not only does the frequency and severity of behaviors decrease, but patients usually also become aware of a decrease in unpleasant dream recall. The mechanism of beneficial effect of clonazepam is unclear, but it may work via reduction of dream-enactment itself rather than restoring REM-related muscle atonia because clonazepam does not normalize abnormal muscle augmentation during REM sleep.[68,70] One drawback of clonazepam is the potential for side effects, including cognitive impairment and falls, especially in elderly patients with neurodegenerative diseases. It should be cautiously adjusted in RBD patients who also have OSA.

Melatonin (3–12 mg at bedtime or 30 minutes before bedtime) has been shown to effective in RBD patients.[71–73] A small randomized controlled trial of exogenous melatonin showed good effectiveness with significantly a reduced number of RWA epochs.[65] Melatonin can be useful when RBD is associated with neurodegenerative diseases with severe dementia such as advanced LBD or motor dysfunction with potential falls. The mechanism of melatonin in RBD is not well understood, although it has been speculated that it restores circadian modulation of REM sleep.[71]

Other medications that may be considered to treat RBD include pramipexole, levodopa, paroxetine, and acetylcholinesterase inhibitors (donepezil and rivastigmine). Compared with clonazepam and melatonin, the total number of studies or subjects using these drugs is small. Therefore, recent standards of practice for the treatment of RBD created by American Academy of Sleep Medicine can be helpful as a comprehensive reference.[67] Efficacy studies of pramipexole, levodopa, and paroxetine have shown contradictory results and anecdotal case reports have demonstrated that these drugs can cause RBD. Because RBD is not a homogeneous clinical entity and because any patient with iRBD has the significant possibility of developing a synucleinopathy, treatment should be personalized according to which diseases and conditions may develop in the future.

CONSIDERATION OF IRBD AS A PRECLINICAL STATE OF NEURODEGENERATIVE DISEASES

Since Braak and colleagues[54] put forward a hypothesis about the development of PD in 2003, there have been accumulating data indicating that various non-parkinsonian features can precede the onset of motor symptoms of PD (or pathologic Lewy body diseases), and these early markers of PD were also demonstrated in apparent iRBD patients. Reported abnormal findings in patients with iRBD that are in common with PD include subtle parkinsonism,[74] anosmia or dysosmia,[74–76] and impaired color discrimination.[74] Neuropsychological abnormalities are visuospatial constructional dysfunction, altered visuospatial learning,[77] executive dysfunction, memory impairment,[78] and impaired facial expression recognition.[79] As for abnormalities in visuospatial constructional abilities and visuospatial learning, they are more likely interpreted as reflecting the preclinical state of LBD.[77]

Physiologic investigations have noted impaired cardiac autonomic activity during wakefulness,[80] decreased heart rate variability following EEG-defined arousals from sleep with or without periodic leg movements detected by PSG,[81] and stable heart and respiration rate during REM sleep that should be more variable than during NREM sleep.[82] These autonomic abnormalities may be seen in patients with MSA, but are not specific for PD.

Functional imaging studies have been conducted with the aim of comparing the findings of iRBD patients with control subjects and/or PD patients. One study using dihydrotetrabenazine positron emission tomography (PET) showed decreased striatal dopaminergic innervation, that suggests a reduced number of dopaminergic substantia nigra neurons.[83] Two other studies used single-photon emission computed tomography (SPECT). One study reported reduced striatal dopamine transporters (the values were between those of controls and PD patients) and similar postsynaptic dopaminergic D2 receptors. This finding places iRBD on the continuous spectrum from normal to PD.[84] The other study showed increased perfusion in the pons and putamen bilaterally and seems to have a similar anatomic metabolic distribution of PD.[85] However, no studies have addressed longitudinal changes by functional neuroimaging in patients with iRBD.

Cardiac ^{123}I-metaiodobenzylguanidine (MIBG) imaging has been used for the early diagnosis of PD because it is now widely accepted that the loss of sympathetic nerve terminals in the heart—interpreted as reduced MIBG uptake—occurs before the deposition of α-synuclein pathology in the central nervous system. To be precise, reduced MIBG uptake is not specific for PD, but may be present in patients with LBD or pure autonomic failure. Decreased cardiac MIBG uptake that was similar to the reduction seen in PD or LBD was also reported in patients with iRBD.[86–88]

Autopsy data about iRBD is available in only two cases. The first was on a patient with a 20-year history of RBD with no cognitive or motor dysfunction throughout the course.[89] The second patient had 15-year history of RBD with no cognitive or neurologic findings.[90] Both patients received a pathologic diagnosis of incidental Lewy body disease. Considering these findings, some investigators take the position that iRBD does not exist and that "cryptogenic RBD" is a more appropriate nosology classification.[91,92]

RBD patients could benefit from neuroprotective treatment if we were able to identify the subgroup of patients who have the highest likelihood to present with motor and/or cognitive dysfunction in the future, and ultimately predict how many years it would take before the onset of synucleinopathies. A recent prospective study suggested that changes in olfaction and color vision might function as a tool for predicting impending neurodegenerative diseases.[93] However, this kind of study is still limited and, in the real world, the clinical course of iRBD varies.[39,40] At present we are not able to make good predictions about the evolution of iRBD. Longitudinal prospective studies to test potential markers among a spectrum of symptoms, signs, and investigations are warranted.

SUMMARY

RBD is an intriguing disorder (1) for sleep researchers as a window to investigate the mechanism of human REM sleep and dream experience, (2) for sleep specialists as a challenging and rewarding clinical process to make a proper diagnosis that includes the background disease or condition, (3) for sleep specialists to develop tailor-made management for the patient and bed partner or family members to improve quality of life of all the involved people, and (4) so sleep specialists consider possible future development of neurodegenerative diseases in the case of iRBD. Neurologists or movement disorder specialists might identify patients presenting with early symptoms of motor disturbance and/or cognitive impairment with yet unconfirmed diagnosis who may not spontaneously complain about minimal nocturnal behaviors. Knowledge about RBD is helpful to reach a correct diagnosis, especially when LBD is suspected.[94] In clinical settings, it is important to closely follow up with patients to look for any changes in the domain of sleep, motor, cognitive, motor, and autonomic functions, as well as psychosocial status.

REFERENCES

1. American Academy of Sleep Medicine. The International classification of sleep disorders. Diagnostic and coding manual. 2nd edition. Westchester (IL): American Academy of Sleep Medicine; 2005. p. 148–52.

2. Boeve BF, Silber MH, Saper CB, et al. Pathophysiology of REM sleep behaviour disorder and relevance to neurodegenerative disease. Brain 2007; 130:2770–88.

3. Iranzo A, Santamaria J, Tolosa E. The clinical and pathophysiological relevance of REM sleep behavior disorder in neurodegenerative diseases. Sleep Med Rev 2009;13:385–401.

4. Ohayon MM, Caulet M, Priest RG. Violent behavior during sleep. J Clin Psychiatry 1997;58:369–76.

5. Chiu HF, Wing YK, Lam LCW, et al. Sleep-related injury in the elderly—an epidemiological study in Hong Kong. Sleep 2000;23:513–7.

6. Okura M, Taniguchi M, Sugita H, et al. Demographic characteristics of RBD patients at a sleep center–with special emphasis on neurodegenerative diseases as the background condition. Brain Nerve 2007;59: 1265–71 [in Japanese].

7. Schenck CH, Hurwitz TD, Mahowald MW. REM sleep behaviour disorder: an update on a series of 96 patients and a review of the world literature. J Sleep Res 1993;2:224–31.

8. Olson EJ, Boeve BF, Silber MH. Rapid eye movement sleep behaviour disorder: demographic, clinical and laboratory findings in 93 cases. Brain 2000;123: 331–9.

9. Schenck CH, Mahowald MW. REM sleep behavior disorder: clinical, developmental, and neuroscience perspectives 16 years after its formalidentification in SLEEP. Sleep 2002;25:120–38.

10. Gagnon JF, Postuma RB, Mazza S, et al. Rapid-eye-movement sleep behaviour disorder and neurodegenerative diseases. Lancet Neurol 2006;5:424–32.

11. Oudiette D, De Cock VC, Lavault S, et al. Nonviolent elaborate behaviors may also occur in REM sleep behavior disorder. Neurology 2009;72:551–7.

12. Iranzo A, Rye DB, Santamaria J, et al. Characteristics of idiopathic REM sleep behavior disorder and that associated with MSA and PD. Neurology 2005; 65:247–52.

13. Schenck CH, Lee SA, Bornemann MA, et al. Potentially lethal behaviors associated with rapid eye movement sleep behavior disorder: review of the literature and forensic implications. J Forensic Sci 2009;54:1475–84.

14. American Academy of Sleep Medicine. The AASM manual for the scoring of sleep and associated events: rules, terminology and technical specifications. Westchester (IL): American Academy of Sleep Medicine; 2007.

15. Frauscher B, Iranzo A, Högl B, et al. Quantification of electromyographic activity during REM sleep in multiple muscles in REM sleep behavior disorder. Sleep 2008;31:724–31.

16. Schenck CH, Boyd JL, Mahowald MW. A parasomnia overlap disorder involving sleepwalking, sleep terrors, and REM sleep behavior disorder in 33 polysomnographically confirmed cases. Sleep 1997;20:972–81.

17. Iranzo A, Santamaria J. Severe obstructive sleep apnea/hypopnea mimicking REM sleep behavior disorder. Sleep 2005;28:203–6.

18. Provini F, Plazzi G, Tinuper P, et al. Nocturnal frontal lobe epilepsy. A clinical and polygraphic overview of 100 consecutive cases. Brain 1999;122(Pt 6):1017–31.

19. Manni R, Terzaghi M. REM behavior disorder associated with epileptic seizures. Neurology 2005;64:883–4.

20. Manni R, Terzaghi M, Zambelli E. REM sleep behaviour disorder in elderly subjects with epilepsy: frequency and clinical aspects of the comorbidity. Epilepsy Res 2007;77:128–33.

21. Jouvet M, Delorme F. Locus coeruleus et sommeil paradoxal. CR Soc Biol 1965;159:895–9 [in French].

22. Sastre JP, Jouvet M. Le comportement onirique du chat. Physiol Behav 1979;22:979–89 [in French].

23. Hendricks JC, Morrison AR, Mann GL. Different behaviors during paradoxical sleep without atonia depend on pontine lesion site. Brain Res 1982;239:81–105.

24. Lu J, Sherman D, Devor M, et al. A putative flip–flop switch for control of REM sleep. Nature 2006;441:589–94.

25. Boeve BF. REM sleep behavior disorder: updated review of the core features, the REM sleep behavior disorder-neurodegenerative disease association, evolving concepts, controversies, and future directions. Ann N Y Acad Sci 2010;1184:15–54.

26. Lai Y, Siegel J. Medullary regions mediating atonia. J Neurosci 1988;8:4790–6.

27. Lai Y, Siegel J. Muscle tone suppression and stepping produced by stimulation of midbrain and rostral pontine reticular formation. J Neurosci 1990;10:2727–34.

28. Shouse M, Siegel J. Pontine regulation of REM sleep components in cats: integrity of the pedunculopontine tegmentum (PPT) is important for phasic events but unnecessary for atonia during REM sleep. Brain Res 1992;571:50–63.

29. Lai Y, Siegel J. Brainstem-mediated locomotion and myoclonic jerks. I. Neural substrates. Brain Res 1997;745:257–64.

30. Lai Y, Siegel J. Brainstem-mediated locomotion and myoclonic jerks. II. Pharmacological effects. Brain Res 1997;745:265–70.

31. Fuller PM, Saper C, Lu J. The pontine REM switch: past and present. J Physiol 2007;584:735–41.

32. Kimura K, Tachibana N, Kohyama J, et al. A discretepontine ischemic lesion could cause REM sleep behavior disorder. Neurology 2000;55:894–5.

33. Plazzi G, Montagna P. Remitting REM sleep behavior disorder as the initial sign of multiple sclerosis. Sleep Med 2002;3:437–9.

34. Zambelis T, Paparrigopoulos T, Soldatos CR. REM sleep behaviour disorder associated with a neurinoma of the left pontocerebellar angle. J Neurol Neurosurg Psychiatry 2002;72:821–2.

35. Condurso R, Aricò I, Romanello G, et al. Status dissociates in multilacunar encephalopathy with median pontine lesion: a videopolygraphic presentation. J Sleep Res 2006;15(Suppl 1):212.

36. Tippmann-Peikert M, Boeve BB, Keegan BM. REM sleep behavior disorder initiated by acute brainstem multiple sclerosis. Neurology 2006;66:1277–9.

37. Xi Z, Luning W. REM sleep behavior disorder in a patient with pontine stroke. Sleep Med 2009;10:143–6.

38. Iranzo A, Aparicio J. A lesson from anatomy: focal brain lesions causing REM sleep behavior disorder. Sleep Med 2009;10:9–12.

39. Schenck CH, Bundlie SR, Mahowald MW. Delayed emergence of a parkinsonian disorder in 38% of 29 older men initially diagnosed with idiopathic rapid eye movement sleep behavior disorder. Neurology 1996;46:388–93.

40. Iranzo A, Molinuevo JL, Santamaria J, et al. Rapid-eye movement sleep behaviour disorder as an early marker for a neurodegenerative disorder: a descriptive study. Lancet Neurol 2006;5:572–7.

41. Postuma RB, Gagnon JF, Vendette M, et al. Quantifying the risk of neurodegenerative disease in idiopathic REM sleep behavior disorder. Neurology 2009;72:1296–300.

42. Claassen DO, Josephs KA, Ahlskog JE, et al. REM sleep behavior disorder preceding other aspects of synucleinopathies by up to half a century. Neurology 2010;75:494–9.

43. Wetter TC, Trenkwalder C, Gershanik O, et al. Polysomnographic measures in Parkinson's disease: a comparison between patients with and without REM sleep disturbances. Wien Klin Wochenschr 2001;113:249–53.

44. Gagnon JF, Bedard MA, Fantini ML, et al. REM sleep behavior disorder and REM sleep without atonia in Parkinson's disease. Neurology 2002;59:585–9.

45. Diederich NJ, Vaillant V, Mancuso G, et al. Progressive sleep 'destructuring' in Parkinson's disease. A polysomnographic study in 46 patients. Sleep Med 2005;6:313–8.

46. De Cock VC, Vidailhet M, Leu S, et al. Restoration of normal muscle control in Parkinson's disease during REM sleep. Brain 2007;130:450–6.

47. Plazzi G, Corsini R, Provini F, et al. REM sleep behavior disorders in multiple system atrophy. Neurology 1997;48:1094–7.

48. Tachibana N, Kimura K, Kitajima K, et al. REM sleep motor dysfunction in multiple system atrophy: with special emphasis on sleep talk and its early clinical manifestation. J Neurol Neurosurg Psychiatry 1997;63:678–81.

49. Boeve BF, Silber MH, Ferman TJ, et al. REM sleep behavior disorder and degenerative dementia. An association likely reflecting Lewy body disease. Neurology 1998;51:363–70.

50. Ferman TJ, Boeve BF, Smith GE, et al. REM sleep behavior disorder and dementia. Cognitive differences when compared with AD. Neurology 1999;52:951–7.

51. Ferman T, Boeve BF, Smith G, et al. Dementia with Lewy bodies may present as dementia with REM sleep behavior disorder without parkinsonism or hallucinations. J Int Neuropsychol Soc 2002;8:907–14.

52. Boeve BF, Silber MH, Parisi JE. Synucleinopathy pathology and REM sleep behavior disorder plus dementia or parkinsonism. Neurology 2003;61:40–5.

53. Boeve BF, Silber MH, Ferman TL. REM sleep behavior disorder in Parkinson's disease and dementia with Lewy bodies. J Geriatr Psychiatry Neurol 2004;17:146–57.

54. Braak H, Del Tredici K, Rub U, et al. Staging of brain pathology related to sporadic Parkinson's disease. Neurobiol Aging 2003;24:197–211.

55. Schenck CH, Mahowald MW. Motor dyscontrol in narcolepsy: rapid-eye movement (REM) sleep without atonia and REM sleep behavior disorder. Ann Neurol 1992;32:3–10.

56. Mayer G, Meier-Ewert K. Motor dyscontrol in sleep of narcoleptic patients (a lifelong development?). J Sleep Res 1993;2:143–8.

57. Dauvilliers Y, Rompré S, Gagnon JF, et al. REM sleep characteristics in narcolepsy and REM sleep behavior disorder. Sleep 2007;30:844–9.

58. Lugaresi E, Medori R, Montagna P, et al. Fatal familial insomnia and dysautonomia with selective degeneration of thalamic nuclei. N Engl J Med 1986;315:997–1003.

59. Lugaresi E, Provini F. Agrypnia excitata: clinical features and pathophysiological implications. Sleep Med Rev 2001;5:313–22.

60. Liguori R, Vincent A, Clover L, et al. Morvan's syndrome: peripheral and central nervous system and cardiac involvement with antibodies to voltage-gated potassium channels. Brain 2001;124:2417–26.

61. Iranzo A, Graus F, Clover L. Rapid eye movement sleep behavior disorder and potassium channel antibody-associated limbic encephalitis. Ann Neurol 2006;59:178–82.

62. Schenck CH, Mahowald MW, Kim SW, et al. Prominent eye movements during NREM sleep and REM sleep behavior disorder associated with fluoxetine treatment of depression and obsessive-compulsive disorder. Sleep 1992;15:226–35.

63. Winkelman JW, James L. Serotonergic antidepressants are associated with REM sleep without atonia. Sleep 2004;27:317–21.

64. Hoque R, Chesson AL Jr. Pharmacologically induced/exacerbated restless legs syndrome, periodic limb movements of sleep, and REM behavior disorder/REM sleep without atonia: literature review, qualitative scoring, and comparative analysis. J Clin Sleep Med 2010;6:79–83.

65. Kunz D, Mahlberg R. A two-part, double-blind, placebo-controlled trial of exogenous melatonin in REM sleep behaviour disorder. J Sleep Res 2010;19:591–6.

66. Gagnon JF, Postuma RB, Montplaisir J. Update on the pharmacology of REM sleep behavior disorder. Neurology 2006;67:742–7.

67. Aurora RN, Zak RS, Maganti RK, et al. Best practice guide for the treatment of REM sleep behavior disorder (RBD). J Clin Sleep Med 2010;6:85–95.

68. Schenck CH, Mahowald MW. Polysomnographic, neurologic, psychiatric, and clinical outcome report on 70 consecutive cases with REM sleep behavior disorder (RBD): sustained clonazepam efficacy in 89.5% of 57 treated patients. Cleve Clin J Med 1990;57:s9–23.

69. Schenck CH, Mahowald MW. REM sleep parasomnias. Neurol Clin 1996;14:697–720.

70. Lapierre O, Montplaisir J. Polysomnographic features of REM sleep behavior disorder: development of a scoring method. Neurology 1992;42:1371–4.

71. Kunz D, Bes F. Melatonin as a therapy in REM sleep behavior disorder patients: an open-labeled pilot study on the possible influence of melatonin on REM-sleep regulation. Mov Disord 1999;14:507–11.

72. Takeuchi N, Uchimura N, Hashizume Y, et al. Melatonin therapy for REM sleep behavior disorder. Psychiatry Clin Neurosci 2001;55:267–9.

73. Boeve BF, Silber MH, Ferman TJ. Melatonin for treatment of REM sleep behavior disorder in neurological disorders: results in 14 patients. Sleep Med 2003;4:281–4.

74. Postuma RB, Lang AE, Massiccotte-Marquez J, et al. Potential early markers of Parkinson disease in idiopathic REM sleep behavior disorder. Neurology 2006;66:845–51.

75. Stiasny-Kolster K, Doerr Y, Möller J, et al. Combination of 'idiopathic' REM sleep behaviour disorder and olfactory dysfunction as possible indicator for synucleinopathy demonstrated by dopamine transporter FP-CIT-SPECT. Brain 2005;128:126–37.

76. Fantini ML, Postuma RB, Montplaisir J, et al. Olfactory deficit in idiopathic rapid eye movements sleep behavior disorder. Brain Res Bull 2006;70:386–90.

77. Ferini-Strambi L, Di Gioia MR, Castronovo V, et al. Neuropsychological assessment in idiopathic REM sleep behavior disorder (RBD): does the idiopathic form of RBD really exist? Neurology 2004;62:41–5.

78. Massicotte-Marquez J, Décary A, Gagnon JF, et al. Executive dysfunction and memory impairment in idiopathic REM sleep behavior disorder. Neurology 2008;70:1250–7.

79. Koyama S, Tachibana N, Masaoka Y, et al. Decreased myocardial ^{123}I-MIBG uptake and impaired facial expression recognition in a patient with REM sleep behavior disorder. Mov Disord 2007;22:746–7.

80. Ferini-Strambi L, Oldani A, Zucconi M, et al. Cardiac autonomic activity during wakefulness and sleep in REM sleep behavior disorder. Sleep 1996;19:367–9.

81. Fantini ML, Michaud M, Gosselin N, et al. Periodic leg movements in REM sleep behavior disorder and related autonomic and EEG activation. Neurology 2002;59:1889–94.

82. Lanfranchi PA, Fradette L, Gagnon JF, et al. Cardiac autonomic regulation during sleep in idiopathic REM sleep behavior disorder. Sleep 2007;30:1019–25.

83. Albin RL, Koeppe RA, Chervin RD, et al. Decreased striatal dopaminergic innervation in REM sleep behavior disorder. Neurology 2000;55:1410–2.

84. Eisensehr I, Linke R, Noachtar S, et al. Reduced striatal dopamine transporters in idiopathic rapid eye movement sleep behaviour disorder. Comparison with Parkinson's disease and controls. Brain 2000;123:1155–60.

85. Mazza S, Soucy JP, Gravel P, et al. Assessing whole brain perfusion changes in patients with REM sleep behavior disorder. Neurology 2006;67:1618–22.

86. Miyamoto T, Miyamoto M, Inoue Y, et al. Reduced cardiac ^{123}I-MIBG scintigraphy inidiopathic REM sleep behavior disorder. Neurology 2006;67:2236–8.

87. Miyamoto T, Miyamoto M, Suzuki K, et al. ^{123}I-MIBG cardiac scintigraphy provides clues to the underlying neurodegenerative disorder in idiopathic REM sleep behavior disorder. Sleep 2008;31:717–23.

88. Oguri T, Tachibana N, Mitake S, et al. Decrease in myocardial ^{123}I-MIBG radioactivity in REM sleep behavior disorder: two patients with different clinical progression. Sleep Med 2008;9:583–5.

89. Uchiyama M, Isse K, Tanaka K, et al. Incidental Lewy body disease in a patient with REM sleep behavior disorder. Neurology 1995;45:709–12.

90. Boeve BF, Dickson DW, Olson EJ, et al. Insights into REM sleep behavior disorder pathophysiology in brainstem-predominant Lewy body disease. Sleep Med 2007;8:60–4.

91. Fantini ML, Ferini-Strambi L, Montplaisir J. Idiopathic REM sleep behavior disorder: toward a better nosologic definition. Neurology 2005;64:780–6.

92. Fantini ML, Ferini-Strambi L. Idiopathic rapid eye movement sleep behaviour disorder. Neurol Sci 2007;28(Suppl 1):S15–20.

93. Postuma RB, Gagnon JF, Vendette M, et al. Olfaction and color vision identify impending neurodegeneration in rapid eye movement sleep behavior disorder. Ann Neurol 2011;69:811–8.

94. McKeith IG, Dickson DW, Lowe J, et al. Diagnosis and management of dementia with Lewy bodies: third report of the LBD Consortium. Neurology 2005;65:1863–72.

Early American Jurisprudence of Sleep Violence

Kenneth J. Weiss, MD[a,b,]*, Elena del Busto, MD[a]

KEYWORDS

• Jurisprudence • Insanity • Parasomnia • Somnambulism

Parasomnias can be considered both mysterious and paradoxic. Actions during sleep can range from simple to complex, raising a fundamental question as to the nature of consciousness, often believed to be a mystery. In addition, these behaviors seem paradoxic, because they seem directed and purposeful and yet occur during a state of relative unconsciousness. One must ask, "What physical actions are possible during a sleeping state?" before judging whether free will was compromised or even absent. Whether those behaviors can be considered purposeful, voluntary, or culpable is a matter for evolving jurisprudence.

Historically, the culpability of actions during sleep followed the Latin aphorism *In somno voluntas non erat libera* (A sleeping person has no free will).[1] Responsibility could not be attached to actions performed during sleep. In ancient times, sleep was considered on the continuum from life to death. Even now, euphemisms and metaphors such as "to be put to sleep" and "the big sleep" refer directly to death. In addition, ancient science considered sleep to be a passive state and failed to distinguish it from other forms of quiescence, such as stupor, intoxication, hypnosis, coma, and hibernation.[2] The Bible refers to sleep as a state of reduced consciousness imposed by God.[3] However, despite this historical perspective on culpability during sleep, to say a criminal defendant was asleep and therefore not criminally responsible sounds naive to the modern ear.

In the nineteenth century sleep was still considered an "intermediate state between wakefulness and death; wakefulness being regarded as the active state of all the animal and intellectual functions, and death as that of their total repression."[4] The jurisprudence of sleep violence was largely reliant on the forensic skills of the attorneys and the folk psychology of the times. The subject was reviewed by Bonkalo[5] in 1974, starting with a Silesian man who in 1791 killed his wife with an ax. The accused argued that he committed the heinous act during a state of sleep-drunkenness (*Schlaftrunkenheit*); he therefore claimed he had no will because he was not fully awake. Noting that the French also acknowledged sleep-drunkenness (*l'ivresse du sommeil*), Bonkalo identified 20 European cases in which a partially awake person was deemed not criminally responsible.

The midtwentieth century marked the modern era of sleep physiology; the advent of polysomnography allowed the detailed descriptions of sleep stages and their behavioral correlates.[6,7] This article reviews how cases of alleged sleep violence were handled by medical experts and jurists in America in the nineteenth century. Our focus is on the formulations of psychiatrist Isaac Ray and the legal scholar Francis Wharton in mid-nineteenth century, followed by an account of a famous 1846 murder trial in Boston. We then examine how closely the older, clinically based formulations conform to our modern views.

The authors have nothing to disclose.

[a] Department of Psychiatry, Perelman School of Medicine at the University of Pennsylvania, Philadelphia, PA 19104, USA

[b] Forensic Psychiatry Fellowship Program, Perelman School of Medicine at the University of Pennsylvania, Philadelphia, PA, USA

* Corresponding author. Two Bala Plaza, Suite 300, Bala Cynwyd, PA 19004.

E-mail address: kenweiss@mail.med.upenn.edu

Sleep Med Clin 6 (2011) 469–482

doi:10.1016/j.jsmc.2011.08.005

ISAAC RAY'S MEDICAL JURISPRUDENCE

Ray, considered the founder of American forensic psychiatry, enjoyed a brief and unsuccessful career as a family physician in Maine before turning his attention to psychiatry (asylum medicine) (**Fig. 1**).[8] While in remote Eastport, Maine, he published in 1838 the first American textbook on forensic psychiatry, *A Treatise on the Medical Jurisprudence of Insanity*.[9] The work, borrowing heavily from the European tradition and case law, became a standard forensic psychiatric text and underwent 4 revisions. Our focus is on the fifth and final edition, published in 1871, which was Ray's final word on sleep disorders and their legal implications.[10]

In his treatise, Ray devoted 4 articles to sleep disorders: "Somnambulism," "Legal Consequences of Somnambulism," "Simulated Somnambulism," and "Somnolentia." With respect to jurisprudence, he is not mysterious in his point of view: "The sleeping state gives rise, in one way or another, to a mental condition in which all moral liberty is destroyed."[10(p521)] The outcome of a nineteenth-century criminal case was based simply on proof that the defendant was asleep at the time in question. Although Ray was a scientist, it did not seem to concern him that there were no scientific tests to distinguish wakefulness from sleep: "What the

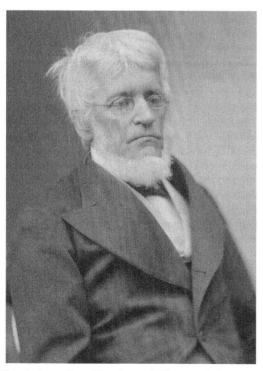

Fig. 1. Isaac Ray. (*Courtesy of* Library of Congress, Brady-Handy Collection, 1865–80.)

essential condition of the brain is in sleep, as distinguished from that of the waking state, is one of the problems of physiology that remains to be solved. The few facts which meet our observation throw but little light on this point, though they serve to indicate the general features of the differences between the two states."[10(p521)] Scientific knowledge of sleep in the nineteenth century, albeit modest at best, required cases be adjudicated. A closer examination of Ray's understanding of sleep states illuminates how criminal cases were viewed.

Somnambulism

Ray questioned whether the sleeping mind represented a continuance of "natural faculties" coupled with the "cooperation" of voluntary muscles. Based on the case presentations provided, along with his interpretation, he notes that sleepwalkers can perform various complex acts. These acts, at times, may look as if the subject is awake, because these movements are performed with such accuracy and precision. In addition, because of the performance of these complex movements, whether the individual is able to see has also been questioned. This factor varies on a case-by-case basis. If a habit is overlearned, Ray implies, it is performed in sleep without the aid of sight. Some individuals defy the understanding of what is humanly possible. The famous somnambulist Jane Rider could reportedly read and write in her sleep. Because Rider could converse in her sleep Ray analogized sleepwalking to dreaming, because dreamers can respond to others within the subject matter of a dream while remaining oblivious to other sounds. In a variant form, cataleptic somnambulism or ecstasis, there is little motor activity, but "the patient converses with fluency and spirit," although usually amnestic for the episode.

Various forms of somnambulism were believed to be a morbid condition, lending itself to the prevailing psychopathologic formulation. Ray hints that ordinary sleepwalking is "a slight modification of dreaming" that is influenced by bodily states. However, ecstasis is closer to epilepsy and hysteria and is therefore associated with insanity. Cataplectic somnambulism can be precipitated by "uterine functions" in women, excessive use of alcohol, or plethora of the blood vessels of the head. Sleepwalking has also been seen in families, and some forms were believed to be heritable, Ray notes.

Ray likens somnambulism to a psychiatric disorder, hinting at a formulation that could have traction in the forensic setting: "In the somnambulist, either the perceptive organs are inordinately excited, and thus he is led to mistake inward for outward sensations; or, the perceptions, if correct, are misapprehended by some obliquity of the reflective powers; in some instances probably, both these events take place. He talks, moves, and acts, unconscious of his real condition and of nearly all his external relations."[10(p509)] In effect, he concludes, the mental derangement in somnambulism is similar to that in mania, although their causes differ. In mania, when patients are restored to health, they regard the period of their derangement as dreamlike, "with grotesque images, heterogeneous associations, and ever-changing scenes." This pattern was sufficient for Ray to consider the emotional derangement in mania and the phenomenon of sleepwalking to share a physiologic pathway.

Ray was impressed that some somnambulists have intellectual powers not present during wakefulness. He discusses Jane Rider, who could sing and play backgammon and imitate others' language only while sleepwalking. Known as the Springfield [Massachusetts] Somnambulist, Rider, as a teenager from Vermont, showed extraordinary behaviors with her eyes closed.[11] Her behaviors, which appeared suddenly, were characterized as paroxysms and, for a while, were associated with chorea. A phrenological examination revealed tenderness over the Organ of Marvellousness.[11] It seems that Ray may have accepted her reputation as a somnambulist at face value, although it is more likely that her mental feats bore little relation to what we would consider a parasomnia.[12]

Legal Consequences of Somnambulism

Ray understood that somnambulism entailed brain disease and, as such, had implications for the reliability of civil acts conducted during sleep. Should the disease be discovered, it raised questions about the validity of contracts and even marriages. Ray implied that the somnambulist has a duty to disclose the condition, lest a contract come under suspicion at a later date. Regarding criminal behavior, he is categorical: "As the somnambulist does not enjoy the free and rational exercise of his understanding, and is more or less unconscious of his outward relations, none of his acts during the paroxysms, can rightfully be imputed to him as crimes."[10(p511)] However, when citing [Johann Christoph] Hoffbauer, Ray suggests that the somnambulist may not be excused fully if, knowing about the condition, he fails to prevent its consequences. Ray is dubious about Hoffbauer's reasoning, namely, that if the somnambulist's acts were considered or planned during waking, there would be no excuse. After all, Ray

says, persons are not punished for their meditations, only their acts. Also noting [François Emmanuel] Foderé, a contemporary of Hoffbauer's, Ray is critical of the notion that because the somnambulist is not delusional, ordinary criminal responsibility applies.

Simulated Somnambulism

In this third of 4 articles on sleep Ray plainly says that somnambulism may be simulated or feigned and then discusses clinical parameters for discovering this type. The 2 principal dynamics are doing something one would not attempt normally and to avoid punishment; this combination is what we now call malingering.

How does one determine whether sleepwalking is simulated? Ray first says, if one can obtain minute details of the behavior in question, it can be compared with the paroxysms of genuine, gold standard cases. A simulator is likely to make mistakes in one way or another. In genuine cases, Ray notes, it would not be possible to explain the individual's behaviors never attempted during waking, unless there had been a systematic attempt to conceal these qualities. Sometimes a simulator can be exposed by a simple procedure such as bandaging the eyes to see if the actions are reproduced. Unfortunately for scientific purposes, in most instances there are no witnesses; therefore the proof of the condition rests on the person's own testimony. If the proof fails to be sufficient, the individual must be held accountable, because, "[O]nce acquit a criminal on the score of somnambulism which is imperfectly or at best but plausibly proved, and it will soon become a favorite excuse for crime, whenever the offender possesses the requisite address for maintaining the deception."[10(p516)] To Ray, the best test of accountability seemed to be in the relationship of the criminal acts to the individual's character and disposition; for example, whether there was a known motive and whether the defendant's assertions seem open and sincere.

Somnolentia

Somnolentia, or sleep-drunkenness, was the nineteenth-century term for a partial awakening during sleep. Ray describes the putative physiology: when one falls asleep, the organs of awareness, one after another, cease to function; and in awakening, they resume working until fully functional. If the waking process is interrupted, by a loud noise or attempts to rouse the sleeper, "the mind does not readily resume its proper relations, misapprehending the impressions made on the senses, and acting accordingly. The mind is then in a state of temporary delirium…sleep-drunkenness. Deceived by false images and unable to reason correctly, the sleeper may commit some deed of violence that shocks no one more than himself when he becomes fully awake."[10(p522)]

Ray devoted a paragraph to the Silesian ax-murder case, noted earlier in Bonkalo's review.[5] The accused, Bernard Schimaidzig, was aroused from sleep to see what he perceived as a phantom. After calling out for a response and receiving none, he picked up a hatchet and attacked. The blow caused a sound that fully awoke him, at which point he discovered he had slain his wife. Witnesses saw Schimaidzig trembling and agitated, crying, "My God my God, what have I done!" The Criminal College of Upper Silesia concluded that the act was committed during the transition between dreaming and wakefulness and found him not responsible.

A more recent example comes from Germany in 1839. This story was quoted by Wharton in his monograph on mental unsoundness[13] and repeated by Ray. A father and son returning from a hunting trip brought their respective firearms to their bedrooms. In the middle of the night, the father jarred the door to the son's room open and the son sprang up and shot him in the chest. As the son shot his father, he was noted to have said, "Dog, what do you want here?" and as the victim fell, the young man said, "Oh! Jesus, it is my father!" This example shows the clinical evidence supporting the adjudication of nonresponsibility: (1) the whole family was known to be restless during sleep; (2) the defendant was easily distressed by dreams and would wake before the dreams had fully dissipated; and (3) the defendant stated that he recalled little, concluding, "I must have been under the delusion that thieves had broken in." The medical experts excused him on the grounds of somnolentia.

Although Ray did not think the English courts were as forgiving as the European, he quoted Sir Matthew Hale at length regarding a story Ray did not consider a "proper case of somnolentia" but that had the same outcome as the previous example. Hale relates that "William Levet being in bed and asleep in the night, his servant hired Frances Freeman to help her do her work, and about twelve of the clock in the night, the servant going to let out Frances, thought she heard thieves breaking open the door; she therefore ran up speedily to her master, and informed him that she thought thieves were breaking open the door; the master, rising suddenly, and taking a rapier, ran down suddenly; Frances hid herself in the buttery, lest she should be discovered; Levet's wife, spying Frances in the buttery, cried out to her husband, 'Here they be that would undo us.'

Levet runs into the buttery, in the dark, not knowing Frances, but thinking her to be a thief, and thrusting with his rapier before him, hit Frances in the breast mortally, whereof she instantly died. This was resolved to be neither murder, nor manslaughter, nor felony."[10(pp524–5)]

Proof of somnolentia is often elusive because it is rarely witnessed and often occurs in the dark. Based on the advice from German medical jurist Mende, Ray defined criteria for identifying somnolentia: "It should appear that the person is habitually a deep, heavy sleeper, and awakened only by much shaking and slapping; that, before sleeping, certain things occasioned disquiet, which might not be removed by sleep, and which, consequently, might give rise to vivid dreams; that the criminal act occurred at the time when the person was usually asleep; that the sudden waking was produced by certain specific causes, unless the result of dreams; that the act is clearly indicative of the absence of consciousness and self-possession; that the person, on fully awaking, is astonished at what he has done, and manifests extreme concern and sorrow."[10(p526)] When motives are obvious either by design or opportunity, Ray cautioned, the plea must be regarded with suspicion.

Francis Wharton's "Mental Unsoundness"

Wharton, a prolific legal scholar from Philadelphia, published his *Monograph on Mental Unsoundness*[13] in 1855, which he included in his larger work on *Medical Jurisprudence* published in the same year (**Fig. 2**).[14] Like Ray, he gathered much of his case material from Europe and classified sleep disorders into somnolentia and somnambulism. Wharton begins his discussion with reserve and circumspection: "In the forensic treatment of such maladies each case must depend upon its own circumstances, when it will also be important for the judge to consider whether the person subject to such a disorder was properly aware of it, and of its possible consequences, and able to take the precautions by which those consequences might have been averted."[13(p119)]

Wharton's general formulation of the relationship between sleep and wakefulness is surprisingly modern for 1855. He understood sleep as a continuation of cerebral life wherein the sleeper is unaware of any motor activity. He suggested that in sleep "the intellect is diverted" by changes in the brain activity. Furthermore, with certain morbid conditions complete wakefulness may not be fully restored, resulting in a state akin to intoxication (*Schlaftrunkenheit*), midway between waking and dreaming. He concluded that because

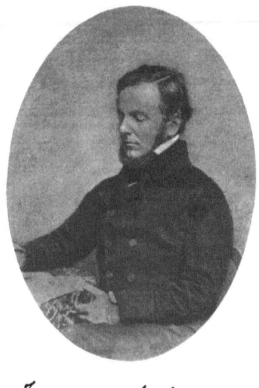

Fig. 2. Francis Wharton at age 34 years. (*From* Wharton HE, editor. Francis Wharton: a memoir. Philadelphia: [self-published]; 1891.)

we are not conscious of dreams during sleep, the same may be said of awareness of one's actions during sleep-intoxication. In such a state, because a person's actions are colored by dreams, one may unintentionally perform acts of violence as if in a dream. In keeping with Ray's view of a sleep-walker's criminal responsibility, he states that "…every act shown to have been committed under its influence is to be disconnected with voluntary moral agency."[13(p120)]

Somnolentia

Wharton's succinct definition of somnolentia is pregnant with its jurisprudence: "Sleep-drunken-ness may be defined to be the lapping over of a profound sleep on the domains of apparent wakefulness, producing an involuntary intoxication on the part of the patient, which destroys at the time his moral agency."[13(p120)] Based on this defi-nition, once the somnolentia has been established, the other critical elements fall into place: the invol-untary nature of the acts at the time and the atten-dant absence of the will. Wharton cites several cases to support his claims. He begins with the description of a military sentry awoken by his commanding officer. The sentry violently attacked with his sword, nearly killing his superior. The expert examinations concluded that the attack was "involuntary and irresponsible." In another case, a man was forcibly awakened and had the instant delusion that a woman in white was carrying away his wife. He attacked and killed the "perpe-trator" only to find that the woman he killed was his wife. Based on evidence of somnolentia, the man was acquitted. Wharton notes that in the United States such a case would be classified as "excusable homicide by misadventure."

Having shown how persons under sleep-drunkenness are not considered responsible for violent acts, Wharton subsequently provides a 6-point test to determine somnolentia (**Table 1**):

When considered in the light of nineteenth-century clinical knowledge, these criteria seem reasonable. The final point is of particular interest because it is a key element of the defense in several recent cases of rape and sexual assault claiming "sexsomnia."[15] The phenomenon of abnormal sexual behavior during sleep is consid-ered a nonrapid eye movement variant of somnambulism. Although this is not a crime when the partner has consented, it becomes a criminal case when not consensual. In such cases, an individual who shows shock at their own behavior and is willing to aid authorities is more likely to be genuine, as Wharton suggests.

By way of contrast, Wharton cites some failed instances of a somnolentia defense. "In the case of *Reg. v. Jackson*, it was urged in defense that the prisoner, who slept in the same room with the prosecutor, had stabbed him in the throat, owing to some sudden impulse during sleep. It was proved, however, that the prisoner had shown malicious feeling against the prosecutor and that she wished him dead. The knife with which the wound had been inflicted bore the appearance of having been recently sharpened, and the prisoner must have reached over her daughter (the prosecutor's wife), who was sleeping in the same bed with him, to produce the wound. These facts are quite adverse to the supposition of the crime having been perpetrated under an impulse from sleep, and the prisoner was convicted."[13(p124)]

Table 1
Wharton's criteria for responsibility in somnolentia

a.	A general tendency to deep and heavy sleep must be shown, out of which the patient could only be awakened by violent and convulsive effort
b.	Before falling asleep, circumstances must be shown producing disquiet which sleep itself does not entirely compose
c.	The act under examination must have occurred at the time when the defendant was usually accustomed to have been asleep
d.	The cause of the sudden awakening must be shown. It is true that this cannot always happen, as sometimes the start may have come from a violent dream
e.	The act must bear throughout, the character of unconsciousness
f.	The actor himself, when he awakes, is generally amazed at his own deed, and it seems to him almost incredible. Generally speaking he does not seek to evade responsibility, though there are some unfortunate cases in which, the wretchedness of the sudden discovery, overcomes the party himself, who seeks to shelter himself from the consequences of a crime of which he was technically, though not morally, guilty

From Wharton F. A treatise on mental unsoundness. Philadelphia: Kay & Brother; 1855.

Somnambulism

Wharton begins this section with a quotation from Benjamin Rush, which has a clear trajectory regarding jurisprudence: "Dreaming is a transient paroxysm of delirium. Somnambulism is nothing but a higher grade of the same disease. Like madness, it is accompanied with muscular action, with incoherent or coherent conduct, and with that complete oblivion of both which takes place in the worst grade of madness."[13(p125)] Wharton proceeds to give elaborate examples, from Europe and America, of sleepwalking behavior. The pattern he shows is that the affected individual gets up, engages in complex behaviors, returns to sleep, and afterwards is amnestic for the event. Such case studies included (1) "Dr. Blacklock, of Edinburgh, who rose from his bed, to which he had retired at an early hour, came into the room where his family were assembled, conversed with them, and afterwards entertained them with a pleasant song, without any of them suspecting he was asleep, and without his retaining after he

awoke the least recollection of what he had done"; (2) a sleepwalking kleptomaniac; and (3) a farmer who, in the middle of the night, ascended his hayloft and thrashed rye until he fell to the floor.[13(pp125–6)] In Wharton's examples, whenever such actions lead to criminal behavior the sleepwalker is held blameless.

Wharton quotes at length the introduction to an article on somnambulism from John Abercrombie's book on the mind.[16] In Abercrombie's formulation, the essential difference between somnambulism and dreaming is how bodily functions are affected. In somnambulism, the mind is not focused on external reality while the body appears to be free to act; consequently, "the individual acts under erroneous impressions, through his organs of sense; not, however, so as to correct his erroneous impressions, but rather to be mixed up with them."[13(p126)] Like Wharton, Abercrombie's examples are of elaborate behaviors accompanied by little awareness afterwards. Wharton cautions about malingered somnambulism, citing a case of a man who set up the situation to cloak an intended crime. He does not explore, however, how one might make the distinction clinically.

THE TIRRELL MURDER TRIAL, 1846

The trial of Albert Tirrell for the murder of his paramour, Mary Ann (or Maria) Bickford, was a newsworthy event in Boston in 1846. The case was a sensation from start to finish because it involved a man and a woman who had left their spouses, a bloody death (a murder or perhaps suicide), a fire, the fleeing of the accused, an unusual somnambulism defense complete with expert testimony, and a remarkable defense attorney named Rufus Choate (**Fig. 3**).

Background

The following facts have been widely published and are extracted from Parker's 1860 *Reminiscences of Rufus Choate*.[17] Parker referred to the Tirrell case as Choate's greatest performance as a defense attorney, amid a storied career as a man with extraordinary oratorical powers. At the time of the incident in 1845, Albert Tirrell was 22 years old and Mary Ann Bickford 21 years. Both had left their spouses and attempted to live together against strong community resistance. Ms Bickford finally settled in a Boston rooming house, where Tirrell is said to have been around the time of her death. The facts of the prosecution included: on October 26, Tirrell was seen in Bickford's room; the house was locked up for the night; at about 4:00 AM, someone in the house heard a noise and then a fall, and a half hour later the

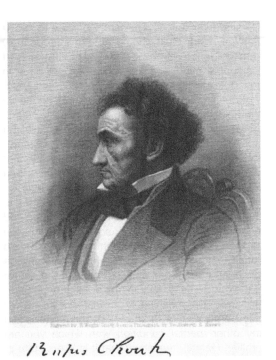

Fig. 3. Tirrell's lawyer Rufus Choate. (*From* Proceedings of the Massachusetts Historical Society, Second Series, vol. XI, Boston, 1896.)

sound of someone leaving; finally, the homeowner heard a groan or cry outside the house and his wife yelled "Fire!" because there was a fire in Bickford's room. The case of murder was established when Bickford was found in her room with her throat cut ear to ear and a bloody razor on the floor. There was evidence that the straw mattress had been set afire with matches. That morning, Tirrell tried to get a carriage ride at Fullam's stable, saying he needed to get away because someone had come into his room and tried to murder him. "His appearance was described as peculiar and wild, and like that of a person in a stupor, when at this place; and the sounds of his voice were like a distressed groan."[17(p221)] Tirrell returned to his home in Weymouth and found his way to New Orleans, where he was arrested months later. Among the reasons he was suspected was that one of the roomers overheard loud conversation between Tirrell and Bickford the evening before. Parker makes the point that public sentiment was predisposed against Tirrell because of a similar case in New York 10 years earlier.

The Government's Case

Tirrell's capital trial for murder began on March 24, 1846 (the arson trial was in 1847). He was represented both by Mr Choate and junior counsel, Annis Merrill, who made the opening statement and examined witnesses. The indictment, published by the *Boston Daily Times*,[18] along with testimony and arguments, accused Tirrell of taking Bickford's life "feloniously, willfully and of his malice aforethought." After jury selection, the government, represented by Samuel D. Parker, presented its opening argument. The prosecutor's statement admitted that the case involved significant circumstantial evidence. Parker went to great length to portray Tirrell as sinful and adulterous. Similarly, he did not sugar-coat the victim's situation. She had left her husband after 2 years of marriage in 1842 and, for a while, engaged in prostitution. While she was living in New Bedford in 1844 she began her affair with Tirrell. The couple had a difficult time establishing themselves in respectable homes in Boston; ultimately they found a "House of Ill Fame" where she used the pseudonym Maria Welch. Shortly after, Tirrell was prosecuted for adultery. As he was about to be tried, his family interceded in the hope of reclaiming him and they negotiated a plea. Only 6 days before Bickford's murder, Tirrell was released on his own recognizance, pending good behavior. The prosecutor speculated that Bickford was afraid of Tirrell and hid. However, he soon found her at the rooming house.

After a recitation of the evidence from the crime scene, Parker called several witnesses, such as the coroner, the owner of the house where Bickford died, firefighters, persons from the stable, and other witnesses. On March 26 the government called to testify a witness named Samuel Head (Heard, according to Isaac Ray). He had seen Tirrell around the time of the incident; however, his testimony seemed to introduce evidence for the defense: "I saw Tirrell in my entry Monday morning between 4 and 5 o'clock; he was talking with my wife in the entry; he appeared to be in a strange state, as asleep or crazy, or as if he didn't know what he wanted; he said he was going to Weymouth, and wanted some clothes that he had left there; he said he wanted to get them, and he appeared so that I was a little afraid of [him] myself; I took hold of him and shook him, and he sort of moved or waked out of a kind of stupor;...when I shook him, he took hold of one of my arms; think he had no gloves on; he seemed much frightened as though he did not know where he was or what he was doing."[18(p14)] On cross-examination, Mr Head continued, "He seemed at the time to be asleep; after I shook him, he said, 'Sam, how came I here[?]' A very few words passed between us after he came out of this state that I have spoke of; it was all one entire observation when he made it; I am now sure that he made the remark about 'Sam' after he was waked up; I told him he had better go to Weymouth, or away."[18(p14)]

The Defense Case

In the morning of the second trial day, Mr Merrill introduced the defense's case to the jury. Tirrell had already been tried and convicted in the press, such that "his cause has been completely overwhelmed with popular odium and prejudice"[18(p17)] (**Fig. 4**). Mr Merrill urged the jurors to disregard the unjust preconceptions of Tirrell that preceded the trial, requesting only a fair hearing. Noting that the government had the burden to prove that the manner of death was murder, Merrill hammered the point that many innocent persons had been convicted on circumstantial evidence. It was still possible that the victim inflicted the wounds on herself, he told the jury. Moreover, no one witnessed Tirrell assaulting Bickford. If the defendant had killed the victim, Merrill said, it was a case of manslaughter: "If it was done in a quarrel—it was not murder, but manslaughter. If it was done in a fit of derangement or accidentally, it would not be pretended that he was guilty of murder. It does not, therefore, follow, that, tho' she might have come to a violent death, by the agency of the defendant, that therefore he is guilty of murder."[18(p19)]

In the afternoon of the second trial day, Merrill introduced the concept of failure of proof as well

THE BOSTON TRAGEDY.

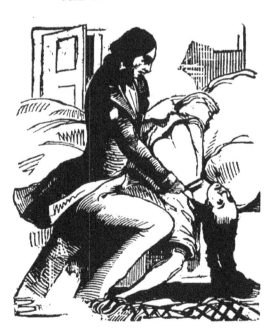

TIRRELL MURDERING MARIA A. BICKFORD,

WHILE IN A STATE OF SOMNAMUBLISM.

Fig. 4. One version of Bickford's death. (*From* The National Police Gazette, April 4, 1846. p. 264.)

as reiterating the government's burden to prove state of mind. Guilt should not be inferred only from evidence of the criminal act, but only if a culpable mind was behind it: "An act done in one state of mind is said to be right; or, at least, not punishable—while the same act, done in another state or condition, becomes a crime punishable by law. The law, therefore, regards the state of mind as a question of *fact*, for the determination of the jury upon the evidence presented before them."[18(p20)] Finally, Merrill suggests that somnambulism is not a rare event and may be well known to some jurors: "And, gentlemen, should any of you be unfamiliar with the state and meaning of spontaneous *somnambulism*—the defense which the defendant sets up in his behalf—should you be satisfied that a homicide has been committed, and that he was the author of the deed—I say, should any of the jury be unfamiliar with the meaning of *somnambulism*—it will only be necessary to show that this state is like any other *mental condition* with which you are familiar. Hence if we show that it is like a state of *dreaming*—like a state of *intoxication*—like a state of *insanity*—yea, more, if we show, as we shall be able to do, that it is a state of real mental derangement—then the case is divested of all obscurity, and is at once rendered perfectly intelligible [italics original]."[18(p21)]

To show the scientific basis for the diagnosis of somnambulism and to set up the defense, Merrill sketches a putative pathophysiology and then calls on contemporary writers and learned treatises: "*Spontaneous somnambulism*, or *sleep-walking*, or *sleep-waking*, as it has been more recently demonstrated by medical writers, is a diseased state of the mind resulting from *certain nervous changes*—which have been known and treated from the earliest periods of antiquity to the present time. It is a mental disease—an unsoundness of mind—and however involved and difficult in theory, — of great familiarity in fact. And we shall show you that it is not only *common*, but that almost every action peculiar to the natural walking [sic] state have been performed by persons in this condition, in ages past, and in our own times, not excepting even the acts of theft, robbery, sacrilege, arson, duel-fighting, and homicide."[18(p21)]

It seems that the attorney was permitted to use medical literature without the aid of an expert witness. Reading excerpts from sources such as Abercrombie, Elliotson, and Ray (not clearly cited), Merrill stated: "There is abundant reason to believe, that a state of somnambulism is a natural to the human constitution—a disease—an actual unsoundness of mind.... With the above agrees every medical authority extent. A condition, as we shall show, far more common than is generally supposed…. Now, suppose this state, which with some persons, is of so frequent occurrence, to be continuous for an hour! Or for five minutes even— that is insanity for the time being; just as real, as thought [sic] it had lasted for an age."[18(p21)] Having said this, and quick to suggest that the defendant had no role in bringing about the condition, Merrill told the jury "that this defendant is one of those unfortunate beings, whom it has pleased the Almighty to visit with this terrible malady."[18(p22)]

The next part of the defense argument was to establish Tirrell's medical condition. The defendant, Merrill said, had suffered from it since age 6 years, often wandering out in inclement weather, and committing acts of violence or mischief. Tirrell would sleepwalk 2 or 3 times a week, and "it was exceedingly difficult to arouse him." More to the point, as an adult having these paroxysms, Tirrell would imagine that he was being pursued by persons trying to murder him. Bringing the clinical history up to date, Merrill cited: "And after he was settled in life by marriage, his malady would some times arise to such power as to cause him to nearly smother his wife in bed. And since he became acquainted with the deceased, this complaint has manifested itself more malignantly than ever. His manner of life has since predisposed his constitution to these states. So much so that he has been known to beat her violently in the states, so that she has made it a subject of notoriety among all her acquaintances."[18(p22)] Suggesting to the jury that Tirrell was aware of the condition, and had adopted some preventive measures, Merrill continues: "[O]n this account he was accustomed to keep a light burning in his room nights, that he might the more easily assist himself to whatever was necessary to remedy these faint or languid turns that followed his sleep waking fits."[18(p22)]

Merrill's entire defense theory was based on failure of proof, with a sleepwalking defense as a fallback: "[W]hile we do not admit that he is the author of this homicide, which God alone can penetrate the mazes of doubt and uncertainty in which this fact is involved, we assert that on that fatal night, we have the indubitable traces that he was in that condition than [sic]; and thank God, we shall produce to you the man who roused him from his lethargy and told him to go home."[18(p22)]

Defense Witnesses

Defense witnesses were called to substantiate what the jury had been told, because attorney Merrill was still in charge at this point. The defendant's mother, Nabby Tirrell, 53 years old, documented the early history of a parasomnia: "Albert has been in the habit of getting up in his sleep since he was four or five years old; once he got asleep, and I left him to go out a few minutes; when I returned, he was gone and I could not find him; he was almost 5… I was in the custom of shaking him to wake him up; afterwards and [when] about 14, he used to try to get up in his sleep, but his brother, who slept with him, prevented it; I know the fact of my own knowledge."[18(p23)] The defendant's brother, Leonard Tirrell, 30 years old, testified that he left home when he was 17 years, and had always slept with Albert. He suggested a progression in the severity of his brother's condition: "I knew his habits of getting up often during the night; he used to when about 10 years old and before; he got up, and I used to get up after him, sometimes he got up, and took hold of me; I was accustomed to shake him and called to him to wake him; he seemed to be gasping at times to make a noise and made a strange noise; sometimes he was want to articulate or talk… I found him once in my room, where I and my wife slept, hallooing; I told him to go back, and was obliged to talk loud and use other means to wake him; he was pale, and said in a spell that persons were after him; he seemed ashamed of it when he woke up;- …he, as well as his mother, took great precautions about fastening the cellar door so as to prevent his falling down cellar."[18(p24)]

On the third day of the trial, the defense called the defendant's cousin, Joel H. Tirrell, 36 years old, who had personal knowledge of Albert's condition and appeared to have no bias. Joel had seen Albert asleep making an "extraordinary" noise, "a noise of distress or agony." Mrs Bickford was there and told Joel to wake him up. She also explained that they kept lamps burning at night on account of the spells of sleepwalking. Joel recalled the pleasant and affectionate relationship between defendant and victim; apparently, Albert was miserable when they were apart. Other witnesses established that the victim, usually referred to as Maria, owned a razor, used to shave her forehead (the fashion of elevating the hairline). There were also several references to the strange sounds Tirrell made during sleep. For example, the defendant's cousin Eben Tirrell (Joel's brother) said the sound was as if Albert was trying to speak. He described it as "a sort of rough catching of the breath, loud and distressing in its character."[18(p27)]

Expert Witnesses

Still on the third trial day, the medical authorities testified. Dr Phinney testified that Bickford's neck wounds were compatible either with homicide or suicide. Dr Walter Channing said that a woman in a high state of excitement could commit suicide with a razor in 1 blow. He had several such cases in his experiences and believed it was the case here. Covering the alternate possibility, Dr Channing said he was familiar with somnambulism and its literature: "In Somnambulism, a person may have the will to act, and yet the moral nature be entirely wanting."[18(p29)] He punctuated his remarks with an assertion that because somnambulism had been scientifically studied, testimony about it could be considered science. He went on to suggest a physiologic dynamic of Tirrell's breathing sounds: "In relation to the noise, in this case it probably is this—that the subject must have slept profoundly, and there has been a short supply of good healthy blood, and the body be thrown into this unnatural state, so that extraordinary efforts must be made to inhale good air into the lungs. Those would originate the noise made by him....I should think [Tirrell] was a somnambulist or sleepwalker, such as I have described."[18(p29)] It seems he was describing a possible case of obstructive sleep apnea. Current research indicates that sleep apnea may be a trigger for somnambulism.[19]

The defense called a prominent psychiatrist, Dr Samuel B. Woodward, superintendent of the Hospital at Worcester (and one of the "Original 13" founders of what is today the American Psychiatric Association). After asserting that he had reviewed the literature on somnambulism and that he had seen 2 "strong" somnambulistic cases and others, he began a discussion of the Jane Rider case and other girls with "paroxysms." After having said this, and without directly linking the phenomenon with the defendant, he stated: "In this somnambulistic state, a person can dress himself, can consistently commit a homicide, set the house on fire, and run out in the street. I think from the evidence in this case, there must be somnambulism.... The moral faculties, as in cases of insanity, are changed and much affected. A person in a state of insanity is dreaming awake, as a somnambulistic is dreaming asleep. They act on false premises, and have lost the regulating power of their minds. They have lost, in such cases, all power of moral distinction."[18(p30)]

Choate's Closing Arguments

On the fourth trial day, defense attorney Choate finally addressed the jury (see **Fig. 3**). His closing arguments lasted all morning and much of the afternoon on March 27. He used a 3-pronged approach: (1) that the injuries to the victim could have been the result of suicide; (2) that there was no direct evidence that Tirrell killed Bickford, thus keeping open the possibility that a third party did it; and (3) that if Tirrell did it, he was in a somnambulistic state. Rather than dwell on the nature of the expert and lay testimony on Tirrell's parasomnia, he repeatedly said that it had been proved. If the jury believed the defendant had committed the murder, they must acquit him: "He is entitled to an acquittal, if he struck the blow on the deceased in an unconscious or not a mentally and morally responsible state or condition of mind."[18(p34)]

Choate immediately switched direction by quoting from "a good old book, which used to lie on the shelves of our good old fathers and mothers, and which they were wanted devotedly to read. This old book is 'Hervey's Meditations,' and I have borrowed it from my mother to read on this occasion."[18(p34)] In part, the quotation he cited read: "Another signal instance of a Providence intent upon our welfare, is that we are preserved safe in the hours of slumber. How are we then lost to all apprehension of danger, even though the murderer be at our bed-side, or his naked sword at our breast! Destitute of all concerned for ourselves, we are unable to think of, much more to provide for, our own security. At these moments, therefore, we lie open to innumerable perils; perils from the restless rage of flames, perils from the insidious artifices of thieves, or the outrageous violence of robbers; perils from the irregular workings of our own thoughts, and, especially from the incursions of our spiritual enemy."[18(p34)] In the afternoon session, Choate opened by recapitulating his insistence that Tirrell was a somnambulist and must be acquitted. He made reference to testimony suggesting that the noise Tirrell made around the time in question was the same type of noise he made during other documented episodes of somnambulism.

Prosecutor Parker argued that the suicide theory was not credible. Furthermore, he stated that no one else at the house could have killed Bickford besides Tirrell. He also pointed out that the defendant had no alibi and that Tirrell had intimated that he was in trouble, explaining his flight. Parker argued that there was no real evidence that Tirrell was sleepwalking during the crime. Moreover, medical experts had stated that individuals waking from this sleep make no sound. He reminded the jurors that it was the defense's burden to prove somnambulism, and that even if such a defense were permitted by law, it had not been proved in fact.

Charge to the Jury and Verdict

On the fifth and final day of the trial, Judge Dewey instructed the jurors that they must decide the manner of death and, if by homicide, whether committed by the defendant. He explained that, because a deadly weapon was used, there would be no consideration of manslaughter, only murder or suicide. In reviewing the testimony on both sides, the judge then arrived at the question of culpability. The jury must decide, he said, if the prisoner was in a state of moral accountability to have committed such an act. Somnambulism is the same as insanity, he told them: "Generally, it is said, that a person in this state, loses some faculties and possesses others. He has no moral control, no reason. Somnambulism is insanity, to be treated as such. If proved, this is a proper ground of defense. Every idle suggestion in relation to this matter should not be listened to; proof of the strongest kind should be required to shield the prisoner from responsibility."[18(p38)] With regard to the expert testimony, the judge warned: "Medical testimony is very properly admitted in these cases, but it should be weighed carefully. It is dangerous to admit the possession of this disease, lest in the reveries of their brains the possessors might commit deeds which in others would be high crimes."[18(p38)]

Judge Dewey concluded his remarks at 10:45 AM and the jury returned its verdict at 12:50 PM. The verdict was "not guilty". The prosecutor demanded that, by law, the jury state the grounds for acquittal. "The Foreman of the Jury stated that the question of Somnambulism had not entered into the consideration of the Jury." Tirrell was discharged from the indictment of murder, and remanded on the charge of arson. In 1847, he was acquitted on the arson charge.

Isaac Ray on the Tirrell Case

Ray devotes about 5 pages of text to the Tirrell case within his "Simulated Somnambulism" article.[10] His sources of information on the facts were newspaper accounts. It seems from his descriptions of the defendant ("dissolute young man") and victim ("a woman more dissolute than [Tirrell]"), that Ray was not sympathetic to the sleepwalking defense. He concluded that the facts of the case did not support a somnambulic state at the time in question.

Contrasting Tirrell's observed behaviors with his history of sleepwalking, Ray writes: "Once in the course of his life he is said to have broken a window and torn down the curtain, and once he went to the table and kicked against the door, saying that he was after a horse. During these seventeen or eighteen years, these were the only exceptions to the general course of the paroxysms; and his friends would not have been likely, under the circumstances, to overlook one. How different his movements on this occasion! He begins by committing murder, and setting fire in the bed and closet. He then goes out of the house, proceeds directly to a stable, tells the people there they must take him out of town as quick as possible; then goes to the Heards [Heads, in the *Boston Daily Times*], wakes them up, inquires for some handkerchiefs they were making for him, and says Fullam is going to take him out of town. Here was not only a remarkable contrast to his usual proceedings in the somnambulic state, but it was just what he would have done had he been wide awake, flying from a terrible scene of blood and fire."[10(pp517–18)] If Tirrell had come to the Heards', it is not consistent that he had appeared coherent at Fullam's stable. Ray argues: "The idea that a somnambulist may continue to pursue the same train of thought and the same course of action, after coming to himself, which he did before, is directly opposed by all our knowledge of this mental condition."[10(p519)] Ray concludes that Tirrell's somnambulism was simulated to avoid prosecution. The key to diagnosing what we would call malingering is that Tirrell did not know how to play out his assumed part of a somnambulist; relying only on descriptions of himself in that state. It seems that Ray, unlike the jury, was persuaded by the circumstantial evidence.

Surprisingly, Ray did not accuse attorney Choate of being disingenuous. In his *Reminiscences*,[17] Parker implies that Choate sincerely believed in his client, principally because the murder lacked motive. Parker considered the popular association of Choate with the somnambulism defense "flippant and unjust." Choate had known Tirrell as a student at Choate's school in Weymouth, and was well familiar with the young man's sleep disorder. Although slightly defensive, Parker asserted: "The credible evidence was in the case and under the eye of a Court not prone to wink at sham defenses or ingenious sophistries. Mr. Choate, relying upon this evidence and the weakness of the government case, triumphantly brought his client within the limits of a fair and legitimate defense. So said the jury of Suffolk; and in this result the Court acquiesced."[17(p227)] Ray suggests that Tirrell's modus operandi was carefully constructed to deceive. Is it possible, one wonders, that he chose Choate (a man with personal knowledge of his somnambulism) to represent him, knowing it would be easier to maintain his charade?

DISCUSSION

The science-based classification of sleep disorders is a twentieth-century development. Although sleepwalking, nightmares, and states of partial awakening were described in antiquity, in the nineteenth century there was a blurring of boundaries between parasomnias and trance states. Collyer[20] reviewed the varieties of altered states of consciousness, noting that certain persons require a specialized state of mind to bring out talents or creative processes; for example, Poe and Lord Byron, who imbibed alcohol before putting pen to paper. Still, the relationship between these self-induced states and sleep is obscure. McNish[4] notes that various substances can induce sleep and seems to accept the prevailing folk wisdom that persons act out dream content. As a devoted phrenologist, McNish reasoned that sleepwalkers avoid anxiety because their Organ of Cautiousness is quiescent. Artificial somnambulism or mesmerism was seen by many physicians as a promising treatment of mental disorders, by exciting the imagination.[21] Yet again, its adherents did little to illuminate true sleep disorders. Some spoke of "lucid" somnambulism, which likely was a form of self-hypnosis.[22] Others placed somnambulism on a continuum with other states and disorders. Exemplifying this is Beard's[23] 1881 categorization of trance states (**Box 1**):

In attempting to tackle the philosophic issues of the will and consciousness, this schema covers much territory within psychiatry and neurology. A person in a trancoidal state becomes an automaton. As such, someone can be trained to start and stop speaking with a mere pinch (**Fig. 5**). It is safe to conclude that, inasmuch as mesmerism was viewed as artificial somnambulism, its study is not relevant to the jurisprudence of parasomnias as defenses to criminal acts. However, today some jurisdictions have permitted a defense of automatism in instances of unlawful behaviors committed in states of partial consciousness.[24]

In America, Amariah Brigham (another of the Original 13 superintendents) corresponded with William L. Stone, Esq. in 1837, inquiring about mesmeric phenomena.[25] It seemed to Brigham that Stone had become a believer in mesmerism. Stone was quick to deny that his interest was cultish or based on blind beliefs, rather on anecdotal evidence. Although predisposed to regard Anton Mesmer, the discoverer of animal magnetism, as a charlatan, Stone became convinced of the phenomenon of animal magnetism through the amazing feats of "somnambulists." It seems that these individuals often put on performances of mental abilities, presumably while in a self-induced state of mental concentration. Mesmerism, like phrenology, fell out of favor by the

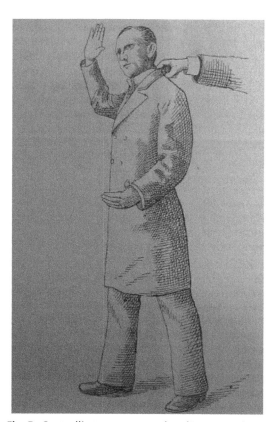

Fig. 5. Controlling a trance speaker. (*From* Beard GM. Nature and phenomena of trance ("hypnotism," or "somnambulism"). New York: GP Putnam's Sons; 1881. p. 20.)

Box 1
Categories of trance states

1. Intellectual trance (absent-mindedness)
2. Emotional trance
3. Spontaneous trance
4. Somnambulistic trance (somnambulism)
5. Cataleptic trance (catalepsy)
6. Ecstatic trance (ecstacy [sic])
7. Alcoholic trance
8. Epileptic trance, or epilepsy
9. Trance sleep
10. Trance coma
11. Trance rigidity
12. Trance lethargy
13. Self-induced trance
14. Mesmeric (artificial) trance

From Beard GM. Nature and Phenomena of Trance ("Hypnotism," or "Somnambulism"). New York: GP Putnam's Sons; 1881.

end of the nineteenth century, replaced by medical hypnosis and the work of Charcot, Breuer, and Freud.[26] Today in American courts, the use of mesmeric phenomena as a defense to crime is virtually nonexistent. However, Waterfield found a small exception in Europe: "In 1879, for instance, a young man, who was a patient of a hypnotherapist, exposed himself in a public lavatory. When his case came to court in France in the early 1880s, he was held to have suffered an attack of spontaneous somnambulism and amnesia, and was acquitted."[26(pp235–6)]

The medical jurisprudence of the somnambulism defense to crime during the nineteenth century was in line with midtwentieth-century thinking. For example, the American Law Institute's Model Penal Code (§2.01) recommends no criminal liability for acts that are involuntary, such as a reflex or convulsion, bodily movements during unconsciousness or sleep, or conduct during hypnosis or resulting from hypnotic suggestion.[27] For lack of better terminology, in the era of Ray and Wharton, nonculpable parasomnic behaviors were conflated with insanity. It is impressive, especially in Ray's commentary, that it was important to rule out malingering. But as we have seen in the Tirrell case, the more troublesome burden is to prove that the criminal act took place during the parasomnic episode.

SUMMARY

Nineteenth-century physicians, legal professionals, and citizens struggled to place sleep disorders in a framework that could illuminate criminal responsibility. On the one hand, there was a popular belief in semiconscious states of mind, ranging from trances to animal magnetism to what we would consider parasomnias. There was no medical research into the nature of sleep and its disorders. The medical experts, for example, in the Tirrell case, based their opinions on historical anecdotes and limited personal experience. Ray and Wharton were concerned about the genuineness of claims made in the service of a criminal defense, with Ray devoting a book article to simulated somnambulism. Wharton's criteria for ruling out malingering certainly ring true today, and were reflected in Bonkalo's criteria in 1974.[5] We believe that contemporary scientific study of sleep phenomena will inform the criminal justice process, in terms of classification, diagnosis, and pathophysiology of sleep disorders., Science can only educate, not decide. Proving the existence of a parasomnia in a sleep laboratory is one matter, but attributing a violent act to that parasomnia on a particular occasion months or years later is another. Correlations are difficult to prove, and judges and juries are skeptical. Even in the Tirrell case, we do not know how the jury would have regarded the somnambulism defense if they considered the defendant to be the perpetrator. In the final analysis, then, criminal cases involving sleep, although informed by science, remain in the hands of citizens reflecting on many factors, just as it was in the nineteenth century.

REFERENCES

1. Schmidt G. Die verbrechen in der schlaftrunkenheit. A. Neur. Psychiat. 176, 1962 as cited and translated into English in Bonkalo A. Impulsive acts and confusion will states during incomplete arousal from sleep: criminological and forensic implications. Psychiatr Q 1974;48:400–9.
2. Dement W. History of sleep physiology and medicine. In: Kryger MH, Roth T, Dement WC, editors. Principles and practice of sleep medicine. 4th edition. Philadelphia: Saunders; 2005. p. 1–12.
3. Ancoli-Israel S. "Sleep is not tangible" or what the Hebrew tradition has to say about sleep. Psychosom Med 2001;63:778–87.
4. McNish R. The philosophy of sleep. New York: Appelton; 1834.
5. Bonkalo A. Impulsive acts and confusion will states during incomplete arousal from sleep: criminological and forensic implications. Psychiatr Q 1974;48:400–9.
6. Aserinsky E, Kleitman N. Regularly occurring periods of eye motility and concomitant phenomena during sleep. Science 1953;118:273–4.
7. Dement W. The occurrence of low voltage fast electroencephalogram patterns during behavioral sleep in the cat. Electroencephalogr Clin Neurophysiol 1958;10:291–6.
8. Weiss KJ. Isaac Ray at 200: phrenology and expert testimony. J Am Acad Psychiatry Law 2007;35:339–45.
9. Ray I. A treatise on the medical jurisprudence of insanity. Boston: Little, Brown, and Company; 1838.
10. Ray I. A treatise on the medical jurisprudence of insanity. 5th edition. Boston: Little, Brown, and Company; 1871.
11. Belden LW. An account of Jane C. Rider, the Springfield somnambulist. Boston Med Surg J 1834;XI: 4–35.
12. Carlson ET. Jane C Rider and her somnambulistic vision. Hist Sci Med 1982;17(Spec 2):110–4.
13. Wharton F. A treatise on mental unsoundness. Philadelphia: Kay & Brother; 1855.
14. Wharton F, Stillé M. A treatise on medical jurisprudence. Philadelphia: Kay & Brother; 1855.
15. Schenck CH, Arnulf I, Mahowald MW. Sleep and sex: what can go wrong? A review of the literature on sleep related disorders and abnormal sexual behaviors and experiences. Sleep 2007;30:683–702.

16. Abercrombie J. Inquiries concerning the intellectual powers and the investigation of truth. Boston: Otis, Broaders, and Co; 1838.

17. Parker EG. Reminiscences of Rufus Choate, the great American advocate. New York: Mason Brothers; 1860.

18. Weeks JE. Trial of Albert John Tirrell for the murder of Mary Ann Bickford, in the Supreme Judicial Court of Massachusetts, holden at Boston, Tuesday, March 24th, 1846. Boston: Boston Daily Times; 1846.

19. Guilleminault C, Palombini L, Pelayo R, et al. Sleepwalking and sleep terrors in prepubertal children: what triggers them? Pediatrics 2003;111(1): 17–25.

20. Collyer RH. Exalted states of the nervous system. London: Henry Renshaw; 1873.

21. Wienholt A. Seven lectures on somnambulism. Edinburgh (United Kingdom): Adam and Charles Black; 1845.

22. Lee E. Animal magnetism and magnetic lucid somnambulism. London: Longmans, Green and Co; 1866.

23. Beard GM. Nature and phenomena of trance ("hypnotism," or "somnambulism"). New York: GP Putnam's Sons; 1881.

24. Schopp RF. Automatism, insanity, and the psychology of criminal responsibility. Cambridge (United Kingdom): Cambridge University Press; 1991.

25. Stone WL. Letter to Doctor A. Brigham, on anima magnetism. New York: George Dearborn; 1837.

26. Waterfield R. Hidden depths: the story of hypnosis. New York: Brunner-Routledge; 2003.

27. Singer RG, LaFond JQ. Criminal law. 5th edition. New York: Aspen; 2010.

Nineteenth-Century Sleep Violence Cases: A Historical View

A. Roger Ekirch, PhD[a],*,
John M. Shneerson, MA, DM, MD, FRCP[b]

KEYWORDS

- Sleep • Parasomnia • Sleep violence
- REM sleep behavior disorder • Medical history

In June 2002, Adam Kieczykowski, a recent student at the Massachusetts Maritime Academy, went on trial for having assaulted, in the course of a single night, 10 female students in their high-rise dormitory at the University of Massachusetts at Amherst. The charges ranged from breaking and entering to 2 counts of attempted rape. Before a Hampshire Superior Court jury, the defense attorney, Raipher Pellegrino, assisted by the testimony of sleep-disorder specialist Mark Pressman, argued that his client had committed the offenses during an episode of sleepwalking and, as such, had not been conscious of his actions. Kieczykowski was said to suffer from a hereditary somnambulistic disorder. Such was his own affliction, testified the defendant's maternal grandfather, that he occasionally tied himself to the bed with a necktie to keep from injuring himself at night.

Remarkably, within 2 hours, the jury acquitted Kieczykowski on all counts. Pellegrino thought that a court ruling to permit the rare defense was the trial's turning point, notwithstanding denials afterward by 2 of the jurors. The judge's skepticism was only allayed when Pressman, dramatically produced the published transcript, of which he owned an original copy, of a Boston trial in 1846. In that case, defense attorneys, armed with medical testimony, had themselves invoked somnambulism to acquit Albert Tirrell, the son of a shoe manufacturer, in the murder of his mistress. The fact that this precedent-setting case had occurred in Massachusetts, Pressman recalls, strengthened Pellegrino's argument in the eyes of the court (Mark Pressman, Philadelphia, PA, personal communication March 25, 26, and June 3, 2010).[1,2]

At no other time are we more vulnerable than during sleep, whether to human malevolence; natural conflagrations like fire; or, literally, to our worst nightmares. Not only are perils often more common at night but our principal links to the outside world, sight, hearing, smell, and touch, are diminished during slumber, if not curtailed altogether. All the more ironic, then, are several medical disorders by which sleepers have themselves been known to inflict violence and even death on strangers, family members, and close friends.

Sleep violence has been an object of wonder for centuries, particularly for legal scholars forced to grapple with the culpability of criminal suspects. As early as 1200, the author of the *Questions de Maître Laurent* observed: "It happens that many men get up at night while asleep, take up weapons or staffs, or get on horseback. What," he asked plaintively, "is the cause of this? What is the remedy?"[1] In the early fourteenth century, the Council of Vienne in Southern France reported instances of murder committed by persons in their sleep, as did the Italian jurist Martinus Garatus Laundensis in the 1400s, a claim repeated in a contemporary Spanish treatise that spoke of "murderous sleepwalkers," "as is well-known has happened in England."[3–5] If so, the paucity of early English legal records, let alone personal papers, such as diaries and correspondence, is of little help. Not until 1686 do surviving documents reveal a likely episode

a Department of History, Virginia Tech, Blacksburg, VA 24018, USA
b Respiratory Support and Sleep Centre, Papworth Hospital, Ermine Street, Papworth Everard, Cambridge CB3 8RE, UK
* Corresponding author. 1901 Pelham Drive, Roanoke, VA.
E-mail address: arekirch@vt.edu

Sleep Med Clin 6 (2011) 483–491
doi:10.1016/j.jsmc.2011.08.007
1556-407X/11/$ – see front matter © 2011 Elsevier Inc. All rights reserved.

involving the death of an officer of the guard and his horse, shot with a blunderbuss by an habitual sleepwalker, Colonel Cheyney Culpepper, brother of Thomas Lord Culpepper, second Baron of Thoresway. After first being convicted of manslaughter by reason of insanity at the Old Bailey in London, Culpepper was pardoned by James II.[3,6] The small number of recorded cases has only accentuated the mysterious nature of disorders associated with sleep violence, rendering our understanding of their underlying dynamics all the more problematic, as has the natural skepticism questioning their authenticity, especially when invoked over the years, albeit infrequently, as a defense during criminal trials.

Patients are typically afflicted by one of several conditions, although it is not unknown for one disorder to overlap with another. Among the most common are sleep terrors (known also as night terrors), occasioned by momentary, frightening hallucinations, resulting in panic and confusion. Episodes, often brought on by stress, occur during incomplete arousal from a deep sleep: non–rapid eye movement (NREM) sleep, which is distinguished by a general absence of dream activity. The individual, often a male child, may suddenly seem to awaken with a gasp or cry, sit up or leap out of bed, and utter nonsensical speech. Beginning in late adolescence and early adulthood, patients have been known to commit violent acts. A related condition is confusional arousals in which persons react aggressively on awakening abruptly from a state of NREM sleep in a disoriented or incomplete condition of alertness. Although just 1% of adults are prone to confusional arousals, it is commonplace among children younger than 5 years of age.[7,8]

Best known today, owing to its sensational character, is REM sleep behavior disorder (RBD), which was formally identified in 1985 by sleep specialists at the University of Minnesota.[9] (**Box 1** lists important events in sleep disorders.) In contrast to other forms of sleep violence, RBD is characterized by vivid dreams, distinguished by their narrative quality, that portray an imaginary person or object other than the unfortunate victim of the patient's aggressive behavior. In technical terms, RBD occurs from the failure of motor inhibition during REM sleep so that muscle tone returns and movements related to cortical activities and dreams mentation takes place. The diminution of motor inhibition, which fails to block messages from the brain to muscles in the body, likely arises from lesions in a small area of the brain stem (ordinarily in the pons or the medulla, which help to regulate physical movement). Individuals have been known to leave their beds, not unlike persons prone to sleepwalking, albeit during a phase, instead, of NREM sleep.[7,9,10]

Box 1
Brief timeline of sleep and sleep disorders during the nineteenth and twentieth centuries

- 1807: Removal of cerebral cortex of birds resulted in sleeplike state (L. Rolando)
- 1814: Publication of *Surprising Case of Rachel Baker, Who Prays and Preaches in Her Sleep: With Specimens of her Extraordinary Performances Taken Down Accurately in Short Hand at the Time; and Showing the Unparalleled Powers She Possesses to Pray, Exhort, and Answer Questions, During Her Unconscious State* by Charles Mais
- 1830: Publication of *The Philosophy of Sleep* by R. MacNish
- 1836: First description of sleep apnea ("Joe" in Dickens's *Pickwick Papers*)
- 1838: Publication of *A Treatise on the Medical Jurisprudence of Insanity* by I. Ray (first extensive discussion of somnambulism as a defense for criminal behaviors)
- 1842: Publication of *The Anatomy of Sleep: or The Art of Procuring Sound and Refreshing Slumber at Will* by E. Binns (also the first book produced by a mechanical type setter)
- 1869: Publication of *Sleep and its Derangements* by W.A. Hammond
- 1880: First description of narcolepsy by J. Gélineau
- 1884: Publication of *Sleep-walking and Hypnotism* by D.H. Tuke
- 1900: Publication of *Interpretation of Dreams* by S. Freud
- 1928: Description of sleep and wakefulness by EEG (Hans Berger)
- 1937 to 1939: Description of characteristics of what would later be called sleep stages (Harvey and colleagues)
- 1953: Description of REM sleep and basic sleep cycle (Aserinsky and Kleitman)
- 1964: First modern sleep laboratory studies of sleepwalking (occurred during deep NREM sleep, not REM)
- 1965: Description of sleep apnea using modern sleep laboratory techniques
- 1968: First use of the term *disorders of arousal* to describe sleepwalking and related disorders by R. Broughton
- 1985: Description of REM behavior disorder by Schenck and Mahowald

The purpose of this article is to explore a handful of instances of sleep violence committed in Great Britain and the United States during the mid–nineteenth century. Although several of these cases have attracted previous scrutiny, others are detailed here for the first time. The few attempts thus far to place sleep violence in an historical context have ranged widely over both time and space. The authors have chosen to focus on a pivotal period in which medical research achieved deeper levels of understanding. The authors' study is confined to Great Britain and the United States, which not only shared a common legal heritage but also drew on a common corpus of scientific research in the early diagnosis of sleep violence. The authors surveyed a large variety of publications, especially magazines, medical periodicals, and newspapers. Electronic databases were of considerable use in the identification of relevant texts, particularly "America's Historical Newspapers," "American Periodical Series Online," "British Periodicals," "Nineteenth Century British Library Newspapers," and "Access Newspaper Archives." These databases allowed us to search the contents of virtually thousands of publications over the span of the nineteenth century.

It is hoped that these episodes will permit a clearer understanding of the history of the disorder and of those who were afflicted by it. No less important is the manner in which families, courts, and physicians grappled with its manifestations in the century preceding its modern diagnosis and treatment.

In early modern Europe, the subject of sleep provoked widespread interest among physicians as well as other members of the educated public. Medical scholars embraced the Aristotelian theory that attributed slumber to a process known as *concoction*. As explained by Thomas Cogan in *The Haven of Health* (1588), fumes arising from the digestion of food in the stomach ascended to the head "where through coldnessesse of the braine, they being congealed, doe stop the conduites and waies of the senses, and so procure sleepe." There was widespread agreement of the benefits of sleep. A balm for both mind and body, it afforded a sanctuary that locked "sences from their cares." In a famous passage, Macbeth speaks of "sleep that knits up the ravell'd sleave of care."[11]

Greater disagreement existed over the nature of dreams. Any number of theories sought to explain their origins, from indigestion to divine providence. As the Stuart poet Francis Hubert reflected: "Dreames are the daughters of the silent night, / Begot on divers mothers." Among all social classes, they, nonetheless, enjoyed widespread currency, every bit as revealing of prospects ahead as of times past. Just a small number of writers denied their importance; and even skeptics were forced to acknowledge a popular preoccupation with nocturnal visions. The author Thomas Tryon wrote in 1689 that an "abundance of ignorant people (foolish women, and men as weak) have in all times, and do frequently at this day make many ridiculous and superstitious observations from their dreams." Only in the eighteenth century, with the growth of scientific rationalism among the literate classes, would dreams become increasingly ridiculed as sources of superstition among lower ranks.[11]

Despite the appeal of dreams, most early authorities seem to have distinguished between nocturnal visions and confused thoughts capable of causing people to commit unnatural deeds in their sleep. Ordinarily, men and women were not held responsible for their unconscious behavior. As early as 1312, the canon *Si Furiosus* had declared: "If a madman, a child, or a sleeper mutilates or kills a man, he incurs no penalty for this."[12] In the sixteenth century, the Spanish scholar Diego de Covarrubias noted: "Such a one lacks understanding and reason and is like a madman." Similarly, Sir George Mackenzie wrote in *The Laws and Customs of Scotland in Matters Criminal* (Edinburgh, 1678): "Such as commit any crime whilst they sleep, are compared to infants ... and therefore they are not punisht."[2] It was always possible, of course, that in some instances Satan, "an enemy," fretted a diarist, who is "alwaies awake," was himself responsible. A seventeenth-century devotion likened the devil at night to a lion pacing back and forth outside a sheepfold. Mental and physical exhaustion, according to conventional wisdom, weakened personal defenses against his attacks.[11]

Apart from scholarly treatises, there is little evidence to suggest the legal outcome of early cases of sleep violence. These writings indicate that acquittals in courts of law were less likely if a defendant could not establish, with the aid of witnesses, a longstanding history of sleepwalking. Then, also, if previous episodes had resulted in violence, the individual had a duty to take proper precautions, such as sleeping alone behind a locked door. Also pertinent was the evidence of ill will between a defendant and his victim before an attack. In sixteenth-century France, a boy was reportedly charged with having mortally stabbed, while still asleep, a schoolmate resting in a nearby room. Not only had the two recently quarreled, but the young offender, according to the story, "confessed to having dreamed that he was killing" the other youth.[13] Least deserving of sympathy, noted the German legal authority Adrianus Beier in *Tractatio Juridica de Jure Dormientium* (1672), was "a sleepwalker," who despite "knowing his condition

… sleeps with an enemy, after a quarrel, in the same house or bedroom and does not put away any weapons. For although at other times he might not be accustomed to take up a weapon on getting out of bed, this will happen more readily with his mind in a violent passion and stirred up by his imagination and fancies he will take up a weapon and kill his enemy."[14]

There is also no doubt courts occasionally concluded that defendants, despite their protestations, had been conscious during an assault. In such instances, the defendant's lack of credibility eclipsed any presumption of innocence attached to the act of sleepwalking. That is, at least, the impression gleaned from the fragments of legal evidence that have survived. "They are not punisht, except they be known to have enmity against the person killed; or that fraud be otherways presumable," wrote Mackenzie. Owing to these concerns, courtroom defenses premised on sleep violence seem, at least in England and its American colonies, to have been rarely used in criminal trials. During the 1700s, not one defendant is known to have invoked such a defense at the Old Bailey.[15]

Only in the nineteenth century did criminal cases involving sleep violence seemingly multiply. This may have been a reflection of the rapid expansion of newspapers and periodicals, both popular and professional, on both sides of the Atlantic. Not only did publications increase in number and frequency but they also gave significantly greater coverage to local news than their predecessors had. During the 1800s, in general, the more intimate and sensational the story, the greater its appeal, particularly for newspapers.[16,17] In 1846, with slight exaggeration, the attorney of a sleepwalker who was charged with murder claimed that the case had "been made the subject of discussion throughout the whole country."[18]

Then, too, victims of RBD and related disorders probably became more apt to invoke sleepwalking as a defense because of its gradual acceptance among both physicians and the public. Beginning in the mid-1700s, somnambulism, as it was widely termed, became a growing object of interest. A New York newspaper, for example, in 1762 described an "Italian gentleman" whose occasional "fits" could only be interrupted by tickling the soles of his feet or sounding a horn in his ears.[19] The renowned Scottish physician, William Cullen, viewed sleepwalking as "an active species of the nightmare," whereas an English encyclopedia attributed the phenomenon to "a very plethoric state of the blood, especially that towards the head; a disturbed imagination, in consequence of horrid dreams; or particular causes that harass

the mind during sleep."[20] More on the mark was a committee of Swiss academicians in 1788 that described the disorder as a "nervous affection, which seizes and quits us during our sleep."[21]

In the United States and Great Britain between 1835 and 1880, the authors have found references to 7 alleged incidents of sleep violence.[3,22-31] Two of the 7 incidents occurred in London, 1 in Glasgow, and the remainder in the states of New Hampshire, Massachusetts, North Carolina, and Kentucky. Excluded from these cases were injuries sustained accidentally by the individuals themselves, whether or not their unconscious intentions were violent. In 1853, for example, having dreamed that he was fighting Indians, a young man in Wilmington, Delaware broke his collarbone by striking not only his bedpost but also a nearby washstand.[32] There is no doubt that there were instances of sleep violence in both Britain and the United States that escaped coverage, as well as occurrences of threatened violence that neither resulted in physical injury nor were ever prosecuted, much less publicized. All that can be said with confidence is that these 7 cases were sufficiently sensational to draw public attention (**Box 2** lists nineteenth century theories of sleep).

Insofar as sleep violence remained a novel defense in the nineteenth century, arguably it was less likely, despite its occasional notoriety, to produce many bogus claims. Among the 7 individuals that the authors have identified, fraud seems probable only in a single instance involving Abraham Prescott of Pembroke, New Hampshire. It is noteworthy that Prescott had already escaped punishment for an earlier episode of violence while

---

Box 2
Nineteenth century theories of sleep

- Passive, inactive, reduced sensory input

  "Sleep is the intermediate state between wakefulness and death; wakefulness being regarded as the active state of all the animal and intellectual functions, and death as that of their total suspension." (The Philosophy of Sleep by R. MacNish, 1830)

- Vascular theories I: blood leaves brain to accumulate in digestive tract

- Vascular theories II: congestive theory (blood goes to the brain causing swelling and congestion)

- Hypnotoxins: accumulation during day and elimination during sleep

sleepwalking. The initial incident, to judge from his medical history and the testimony of his victims, seems to have been genuine. On a winter night in 1833, he left his bed, allegedly in an unconscious state, and struck his master and his wife, Chauncey and Sally Cochran, with an axe while both lay asleep in an adjacent room. The couple, on recovering from their wounds, dismissed the attack as an aberration in light of Prescott's normal behavior. In sharp contrast, evidence pertaining to a second incident 6 months later was probably contrived. Emboldened by his exoneration after the initial episode, Prescott likely pushed his luck too far by adopting the same defense when charged with fracturing the skull of Mrs Cochran, who, it later seemed to a skeptical jury, had rejected his romantic overtures while picking strawberries. Found guilty, he received the death penalty.[22] In light of his earlier exoneration, the Prescott case appears to have been the proverbial exception that proves the rule.

Of the 7 individuals, including Prescott from the first assault, all were adults with the exception of a 17-year-old girl and an 18-year-old boy. Even so, as a group, they were disproportionately young. One was aged 22 years, a second was aged 28 years, and a third was aged 33 years. Another was said to be young. Only the age of Esther Griggs of London remains unknown, apart from the fact that she had 3 young children. Also, most were evidently single, except for Simon Fraser and Albert Tirrell. At least 4 individuals were servants and laborers or otherwise described as poor. For example, Fraser was a saw grinder in Scotland. None of the 7 were described as middle class, much less genteel in their social origins, save for Tirrell, who, "under his father," was "brought up to the shoe manufacturing business" in Massachusetts before allegedly striking out on his own to open a brothel in New Bedford.[24]

The evidence is not so precise as to pinpoint the form of sleep violence in most of the 7 cases. One probable exception, in Nicholasville, Kentucky, was a man named Fain, who, having been threatened earlier in the day by a stranger, was abruptly awakened that evening in a hotel lobby by a porter, whom Fain shot 3 times. Not only did Fain have a long history of troubled slumber, but he had "recently lost much sleep" tending to his ill children.[29] Among modern victims of confusional arousal, sleep deprivation is known to contribute to adult episodes, which, as in Fain's case, normally occur during the first third of one's slumber. As a man, Fain also fits the modern profile, although his age was older than that of most patients today.[7]

By contrast, Sarah Minchin was a likely victim of sleep terrors. The London servant was 17 years old when accused in 1853 of leaving her bedroom and trying to slit the throat of her master's young son. Convicted at the Old Bailey of "unlawfully wounding," for which she was sentenced to 3 months in prison, Sarah had often screamed in the middle of terrifying dreams during her Gloucestershire childhood. "She screams out a good deal in her sleep, and on that account she always slept in the room with me," her mother testified at the trial.[26] Abraham Prescott was given to similar episodes as a child, although his spells, at least according to his mother, "lasted sometimes half the night," whereas sleep terrors today extend at most for up to 10 to 20 minutes.[22]

Sleep deprivation is an aggravating factor, not just in instances of confusional arousal but in most forms of sleep violence. Before the twentieth century, sleep was frequently poor, particularly for the lower orders whose slumber fell prey to a variety of environmental vexations, ranging from noisy streets and freezing temperatures to inadequate bedding, not to mention bedbugs, fleas, and lice. Moreover, whatever one's social class, the quality of sleep today is invariably superior because of the improved medications designed to treat common illnesses and insomnia.[11,33] All 7 individuals, not just Fain, Prescott, and Minchin, were known to have histories of troubled sleep dating to childhood. In addition to restless sleep, episodes of sleepwalking afflicted Fraser from an early age. They also afflicted Tirrell, who, despite inclement weather, occasionally strayed far from home as a child.

Communities seem to have viewed sleepwalkers, those at least with no history of violence either to themselves or to others, as objects of curiosity and amusement. In Davidson County, North Carolina, for example, Click was "quite well known in the neighborhood as a somnambulist."[30] A New York Times essay reflected in 1879: "Happily, fatal results are quite rare - somnambulists, as a rule, preferring to indulge in amusing and instructive eccentricities."[34]

As for instances of past violence, 2 of the 7 individuals, Tirrell and Fraser, had allegedly committed 1 or more acts. For example, before killing his son in 1878, Fraser had once tried to strangle his half sister, assault his father, and, on yet another occasion, dragged his wife from what he thought was a burning house. In response, Mrs Fraser resorted to hiding knives at night "lest her husband should readily find a dangerous weapon." As an adolescent, Tirrell had destroyed a pair of curtains and broken a glass window. Once married, he attempted to smother his wife.[27]

In the 7 instances that the authors examined, the victims of sleep violence included 5 adults and 3 children, 4 of whom died as a result of their injuries.

Four of the 7 assailants thought, in their unconscious states, that they were responding to imminent peril. Fraser, who battered the skull of his son against a wall, dreamed that the boy was a wild beast from whom his family needed protection.[27] Young Click had been hired by a merchant, Uriah Phelps, to join him overnight in guarding his store from "some negroes" who had earlier been ejected. Imagining Phelps to be an intruder in a dream, Click beheaded the merchant with an axe, only to awaken the next morning bereft of any memory of the gruesome crime.[30]

And then there was Esther Griggs' frenzied attempt, in the middle of a dream, to save her 3 children from the flames of an imaginary fire in her upstairs flat. Responding at 1:30 in the morning to cries of "Oh, my children! Save my children," a pair of constables discovered 2 youths huddled in a dark room, and the youngest had just been thrown through a closed window to the street below (somehow, he managed to survive). "I have no doubt," vouched one of the officers, "that if I and the other constable had not gone to the room, all three of the children would have been flung out into the street."[3]

We would be wrong to conclude that medical science in the nineteenth century, despite its deficiencies, failed to address the phenomenon of sleep violence. Medical research advanced rapidly, especially in Britain and Continental Europe. The United States remained Europe's stepchild until the final decades of the nineteenth century, when it joined the ranks of Britain, France, and Germany in research productivity, finally overtaking each after World War I.[35]

Psychiatry emerged as a distinctive branch of medicine over the course of the 1800s, dedicated, along with other fields, to clinical research. **Box 3** contains a timeline of important historical events in psychiatry. No longer did doctors attribute mental illness to nervous vapors, vitiated blood, or to the organs of the body. Professional associations and journals followed quickly, resulting in greater respectability for practitioners. Both asylums and universities in Europe and the United States employed growing numbers of psychiatrists. Now more than ever, their testimony in courtrooms often proved critical to determining whether criminal defendants were responsible for their acts.[36,37]

Although the earliest discussions of sleep violence were confined to legal scholars, by the early nineteenth century, physicians also turned to studying instances of the disorder because of the advances in psychiatry and neurology and the medical profession's longstanding fascination with somnambulism, which the public continued

---

Box 3
Brief timeline of mental health: 1745 to 1899

- 1751: Saint Luke's Hospital for Lunatics in London established
- 1758: Publication of *A Treatise on Madness* by W. Battie
- 1788: Treatment of George III for mental illness
- 1808: The term psychiatry is coined by Johann Christian Reil, a German physician
- 1812: Publication of *Medical Inquiries and Observations Upon Diseases of the Mind* by Benjamin Rush (father of American psychiatry)
- 1821: Lithium was first isolated and described by William Thomas Brande, an English chemist
- 1838: Publication of *A Treatise on the Medical Jurisprudence of Insanity* by I. Ray, influential volume on forensic psychiatry
- 1841: Founding of the Association of Medical Officers of Asylums and Hospitals for the Insane, forerunner of the Royal College of Psychiatrists (England, 1971)
- 1843: Publication of the *Annales medico-psychologiques*
- 1843: M'Naghten rules for determining legal insanity in England following special verdict
- 1844: Founding of the Association of Medical Superintendents of American Institutions for the Insane in Philadelphia
- 1845: In England and Wales, Lunacy Act and the County Asylums Act were passed, leading to the setting up of the Lunacy Commission
- 1853: Publication in England of the *Asylum Journal*; renamed in 1858 the *Journal of Mental Science*
- 1879: First psychology laboratory established in Germany, start of psychology as an academic discipline (W. Wundt)
- 1883: Classification of mental disorders by Emil Krapelin
- 1883: Laboratory of Psychology established at Johns Hopkins (G. Stanley Hall)
- 1890: First publication of *Principles of Psychology* by William James
- 1893: First description of "dementia praecox," currently schizophrenia, by Emil Krapelin

---

to share. Ironically, although the greatest advances were pioneered in Europe, the first medical reference to sleep violence seems to have been in an American translation in 1809 of *Recherches physiologiques sur la vie et la mort*

(1800) by the famous French psychologist Xavier Bichat. Although Bichat himself did not address the phenomenon, the translator, Tobias Watkins, added a footnote to a textual reference to sleep-walking in which he recounted an episode, "known only to few," whereby a "respectable farmer" years earlier had dragged his bed (with his wife still aboard) to place on a hearth, only to leave the farm with a wagonload of produce before returning to bed before dawn.[38]

Sleep violence first attracted serious medical scrutiny in France. At least 2 prominent physicians discussed the condition in their published research: Etienne Jean Georget in his 1825 study (*Examen médical des procès criminels...*[39]) and Charles Chrétien Henri Marc, author of *De la folie: considéré dans ses rapports avec les questions médico-judiciaires* (1840).[40] Georget averred: "A crime committed by an individual in a state of somnambulism should not be regarded as a voluntary act." On the other hand, he acknowledged the difficulty of confirming the existence of the disorder, particularly in the presence of a "probable cause" that "naturally" explained "the criminal act." It was, in his judgment, "up to judges and juries to assess the circumstances" of each case. For Marc, an offense committed during an episode of sleepwalking was no more culpable than a temporary act of insanity, although, like Georget, he recognized the potential for chicanery.

By the 1840s, well-known English psychiatrists, like John MacMichan Pagan and Forbes Winslow,[3,41,42] included references to sleep violence in their own studies. To judge from these and subsequent publications, physicians viewed the phenomenon as a genuine disorder, a consequence of sleepwalking in which a very small number of patients resorted to violence in a state of unconsciousness. Although ambivalent about the ability of physicians to determine criminal responsibility, Pagan, for instance, wrote in *The Medical Jurisprudence of Insanity* (1840): "Nevertheless, it is a real affection, and must not altogether be disregarded by the medical jurist." He also addressed episodes of violence known to accompany night terrors and confusional arousals: "When a person is awoke by a frightful dream, or by some extraordinary cause, either internal or external, he may, perhaps, commit murder, before he has recovered the full possession of his senses."

In criminal trials, physicians often drew on their professional experience. Although their exposure to the disorder was limited, they extrapolated from instances of somnambulism in theorizing about patients' capacity for causing physical injury. As a consequence, not just medical studies but their own testimony served to broaden awareness among other physicians. For example, during Prescott's trial in 1833, Rufus Wyman, MD, the superintendent of the McLean Asylum for the Insane near Boston, testified that he himself had known "two or three cases of somnambulism," whereas another physician described "a remarkable case" in Maine whereby the patient had attempted to hang himself from the limb of a tall tree (fortunately he tied the rope to his feet).[22]

More ambitious was the defense mounted 13 years later on behalf of Albert Tirrell during his trial in Boston. Tirrell had allegedly slashed the throat of his mistress. His defense, assured his attorney, "would be sustained by some of the most distinguished medical men in the country, who have treated persons in this state, and who will speak from experience as well as theory." Three doctors testified to the nature of sleepwalking, with one, Walter Channing, citing studies by more than a half-dozen authorities. "The difference between somnambulism and dreaming," he declared, "is sleep with walking in the first instance and sleep without walking in the other." As for the possibility of violence, "The individual," he noted, "may do acts, from which, in a waking state, he would shrink with horror." A "waking dream with the regulating power absent," echoed the superintendent of the Lunatic Hospital at Worcester. Channing also cited the incident in which Cheyney Culpepper, in 1686, "in a fit of somnambulism shot a soldier of the horse-guards." "This subject is an old one," he informed the court, "not a new one."

Not that medical testimony, whatever the source or quality, always swayed jurors. Pagan, in *The Medical Jurisprudence of Insanity*, feared that "it would be exceedingly difficult to persuade a jury of the real existence of such a condition." Just 4 years earlier, Prescott, given the inherent weakness of his case, was found guilty and hanged. The foreman of the Tirrell jury later claimed that jurors had not even weighed the evidence of sleepwalking; they had instead returned a verdict of innocent because the prosecution had failed to prove its case, thus, causing a writer for the *Boston Daily Mail* to reflect: "This fact only shows how different are the estimates of the weight of evidence among men."[18] All the same, expert testimony increasingly benefited defendants, especially if a history of sleepwalking could be established or, more importantly, a prior pattern of violence during episodes of somnambulism. In Great Britain, both Esther Griggs in 1859 and Simon Fraser in 1878 were set free after the presentation of extensive medical testimony. In Kentucky in 1879, Fain was initially convicted of manslaughter, but the state court of appeals overturned the verdict principally on the grounds that he had not been allowed to "prove by medical experts that persons asleep sometimes act as if awake." As the appellate court observed in its opinion: "The writings of medical and medico-legal authors contain accounts of many well-authenticated cases in which homicides have been committed while the perpetrator was either asleep or just being aroused from sleep."[29]

Not for another century would researchers determine the underlying causes of sleep violence or devise effective courses of treatment. A writer reflected soon after the Fraser trial in Scotland: "This propensity to sleep-walking is a curious phenomenon and has attracted a good deal of attention from men of science; but, unfortunately, no cure has as yet been discovered for the disease."

Still and all, nineteenth-century physicians were the first to distinguish genuine disorders from what had previously been little more than legal curiosities: medical disorders capable of absolving men and women of responsibility for violence that might otherwise have sent them to prison or the gallows. To be sure, as Albert Tirrell's attorney declared, sleep violence was not a new story. A small number of legal scholars had been aware of the phenomenon for centuries. But owing in large measure to well-publicized trials, like Tirrell's (ending in his acquittal), legal precedents were set and psychiatric knowledge advanced, by fits and starts, in Great Britain and the United States.

ACKNOWLEDGMENTS

Many thanks to Mark Pressman and Carlos Schenck for their assistance.

REFERENCES

1. Contrada, Fred, Man, 19, acquitted of assaults in Dorm, 2002. Available at: www.masslive.news. Accessed June 8, 2010.
2. Beal B. Northampton (MA): Daily Hampshire Gazette. June 25, 2002.
3. Walker N. Crime and insanity in England. Edinburgh (United Kingdom): Edinburgh University Press; 1968.
4. Communication from Jonathan Woolfson. East Lansing (MI): H-Albion; 1997.
5. Crusius, Andreas J. De nocte et nocturnis officiis, tam sacris, quam prophanis, lucubrationes historico-philologico-juridicae. Bremen (Germany): Köhlerus; 1660.
6. Unknown to John Fenwick. ADM 77/3. Kew (England): National Archives; 1686/87.
7. Shneerson JM. Sleep medicine: a guide to sleep and its disorders. Oxford (United Kingdom): Blackwell; 2005.
8. Ohayon M, Guilleminault C, Priest RG. Night terrors, sleep-walking, and confusional arousals in the general population: their frequency and relationship to other sleep and mental disorders. J Clin Psychiatr 1999;60:268–76.
9. Schenck CH. Sleep: a groundbreaking guide to the mysteries, the problems, and the solutions. New York: Penquin; 2007. p. 198–200.
10. Dement WC, Vaughan C. The promise of sleep. New York: Delacorte; 1999.
11. Ekirch AR. At day's close: night in times past. New York: Norton; 2005.
12. Verdon J. Night in the Middle Ages, George Holoch, trans. Notre Dame (IN): University of Notre Dame Press; 2002.
13. Joubert L. Treatise on laughter, Gregory David De Rocher, trans. University, Al. Tuscaloosa (AL): University of Alabama Press; 1980.
14. Beier A. Tractatio juridica de jure dormientium. Magdeburg (Germany): Hendel; 1726.
15. The Proceedings of the Old Bailey, 1674–1913. Available at: http://www.oldbaileyonline.org. Accessed September 29, 2009.
16. Lehuu I. Carnival on the page: popular print media in antebellum America. Chapel Hill (NC): University of North Carolina Press; 2000.
17. Barker H. Newspapers, politics, and English society, 1695–1855. Harlow (England): Longman; 2000.
18. Trial of Albert Tirrell, for the murder of Mrs. Maria A. Bickford. Boston: H.B. Skinner; 1846.
19. A remarkable story of a gentleman walking in his sleep. New York: Mercury; 1762.
20. Willich AF. The domestic encyclopaedia; or, a dictionary of facts, and useful knowledge, 4. London: Murray and Highle; 1802. p. 79–80.
21. A true and surprising account of a natural sleepwalker, read before the philosophical society of Lausanne in Switzerland, on the 6th of 1788. Edinburgh (United Kingdom): Peter Hill; 1792.
22. Report of the trial of Abraham Prescott for the murder of Mrs. Sally Cochran, of Pembroke, 1833. Manchester (NH): Daily Mirror; 1869.
23. Evidences of insanity. Boston Med Surg J 1835;11:23.
24. Trial of Albert John Tirrell. Rural repository devoted to polite literature. Hudson (NY): 1846;1:13.
25. Natural somnambulism. Boston Med Surg J 1846; 34:10.
26. The proceedings of the Old Bailey, 1674–1913. 1853, # 725 [Sarah Minchin]. Available at: http://www.old-baileyonline.org. Accessed September 29, 2009.
27. Yellowless D. Homicide by a somnambulist. Br J Psychiatry 1878;24:451–8.
28. Kentucky court of appeals. Central Law J 1880;10:4.
29. Fain V. The commonwealth, court of appeals of Kentucky; 1879.
30. Killed in his sleep. New York City: National Police Gazette; 1880;36:5.

31. Bonkalo A. Impulsive acts and confusional states during incomplete arousal from sleep: criminological and forensic implications. Psychiatr Q 1974;48:400–9.

32. Warlike in his sleep. The Sun (Baltimore); 1853.

33. Weisman RJ. Night in America: staying awake, sleeping and dreaming from colonial to modern times [Phd dissertation]. New York City: Columbia University; 2008.

34. Somnambulism. New York City: New York Times; 1879.

35. Numbers RL, Warner JH. The maturation of American medical science. In: Leavitt JW, Numbers RL, editors. Sickness and health in America. Madison (WI): University of Wisconsin Press; 1997. p. 130–42.

36. Shorter E. A history of psychiatry: from the era of the asylum to the age of Prozac. New York: John Wiley; 1997. p. 69–71.

37. Porter R. Madness: a brief history. Oxford (United Kingdom): Oxford University Press; 2002. p. 153–5.

38. Bichat X. Physiological researchers upon life and death, Tobias Watkins, trans. Philadelphia: Smith & Maxwell; 1809.

39. Georget EJ. Examen médical des procès criminels. Paris (France): Migneret; 1825.

40. Marc CCH. De la folie: considéré dans ses rapports avec les questions médico-judiciaires, vol. 2. Paris (France): J.-B. Bailliere; 1840.

41. Pagan JM. The medical jurisprudence of insanity. London: Ball, Arnold & Co; 1840.

42. Winslow F. The plea of insanity in criminal cases. London: Da Cap; 1843 [reprint, New York; 1983].

The Clinical Features of Sleep Violence in Arousal Disorders: A Historical Review

John M. Shneerson, MA, DM, MD, FRCP[a],*,
A. Roger Ekirch, PhD[b]

KEYWORDS

- Sleep • Parasomnia • Sleep violence
- REM sleep behavior disorder • Medical history

Sleep is characterized by a state of reduced awareness and responsiveness to stimuli; nevertheless, a wide range of physical activities is recognized to take place during sleep. These activities include not only common behaviors such as sleepwalking and sleeptalking, but also violent activities that may lead to injury to the sleeper, the bed partner, or another person nearby. There are, however, remarkably few data regarding the details of what occurs during these violent episodes, and any data available come only from individual case reports and short series.

The authors have examined the historical literature to characterize the features of sleep violence more precisely, and to relate these events to the modern understanding of the underlying neurologic abnormalities during non–rapid eye movement (REM) sleep arousal disorders.

METHODS

The reports examined in this article were identified from sources that span the past 500 years up to the 1990s. Most, however, were published in the United States and Great Britain during the last 2 centuries. Sources included medical books, court transcripts, newspapers, and periodicals. The degree of detail of the descriptions of the events varied, but most gave sufficient information to indicate that the cause was an arousal disorder. The information abstracted included the age and gender of the person involved, the type of activity, particularly to whom the violence was directed, the implement used, nature of the attack, evidence for any recall, emotional expression during the episode, any trigger factors for the event, responsiveness to the environment, and premeditation of the attack.

RESULTS

Twenty-four articles were identified, which included reports of 45 individuals. Several publications included more than one case history and several individuals were reported in more than one publication. The ages were available for 13 of the subjects, who were all between 17 and 35 years old. Three others were described as "young" or "a schoolboy." Forty of the subjects were male and only 5 were female. A selection of illustrative brief case histories is given in **Box 1**. The most important features of these events fell into the following categories.

Motor Activities

In several reports the frenetic aspects of the violence were emphasized.[1,4,5] The violence was sometimes inaccurately directed,[6,7] but in other

Funding support: Nil.

The authors have nothing to disclose.

[a] Respiratory Support and Sleep Centre, Papworth Hospital, Ermine Street, Papworth Everard, Cambridge CB23 3RE, UK

[b] Department of History, Virginia Tech, Blacksburg, VA 24018, USA

* Corresponding author.

E-mail address: john.shneerson@papworth.nhs.uk

Sleep Med Clin 6 (2011) 493–498

doi:10.1016/j.jsmc.2011.08.004

Box 1
Selected case histories

Simon Fraser, 28-year-old laborer, was aware at 1.00 AM of a wild beast on his bed attacking his child. He dashed his son, aged 18 months, against the wall and killed him. Surprise and remorse afterwards.[1]

Bernard Schidmaizig of Siberia heard a noise at midnight, saw a shape, picked up an axe, and killed his wife.[2]

Robert Ledru, a detective, was holidaying in Le Havre while recovering from a nervous breakdown from solving a complex case. He was called in to help the local police following a murder on the beach at night. His examination of the footprints in the sand and the bullet led him to conclude correctly that he had committed the murder while sleepwalking, although he had no recollection of this.[3]

A lay teacher entered the room of one of the brothers carrying scissors. The brother jumped out of bed and the sleepwalker then attacked the mattress 3 or 4 times with his scissors. He had no recollection of this the next morning.[4]

John Cooke, Civil Engineer in Denver, Colorado stabbed himself 4 times in his sleep and bled to death. Just before he died he related to his wife a dream of being surrounded by enemies trying to ruin him, and finally an evil spirit persuaded him to kill himself. He slept through the violence and the intense pain that it would have caused if he had been awake.[3]

Uriah Phelps employed O.W. Click, a young man known as a sleepwalker, to protect him after a disturbance at night. Click picked up an axe near where they slept and cut Uriah Phelps' head off. At daybreak he awoke and raised the alarm, and the neighbors found that the trunkless head had rolled some distance from the rest of the body and was mutilated and gashed. Click had no recollection of the event and had been on friendly terms with the deceased.[5]

---

cases, such as those victims who were killed by gunshot,[2,3,8] it required considerable precision.

The target of the violence in some cases was imaginary,[6,9,10] and this situation arose particularly while the subject was sleepwalking. There were 2 reports of an empty bed being attacked.[4,11] Two subjects caused self harm[3,6] and one of these episodes had a fatal outcome.[3] In most cases the violence was directed against the bed partner,[2,3,7,12–14] or occasionally against a child[1–3] or the subject's mother.[15] The proximity of the victim to the aggressor was emphasized in several reports,[5,12,16,17] although in others the subject sleepwalked before being violent.[3,6,9,12,18] In two incidents nearby animals, including a horse, were attacked.[2,7]

In a few cases no weapon was used, such as when a baby was thrown out of a window[2] or a child's head dashed against a wall,[1] or the partner strangled.[12] In the other reports the method of committing violence reflected the availability of nearby potential weapons. Implements included razors,[17] knives,[2,3,11,12,15,19,20] daggers,[18] a sword,[16,21] scissors,[4] axes,[2,5,7,12] a hammer,[12] shovel,[13] a bayonet,[12] and guns.[2,3,8]

A feature of the violence was that repetitive injuries were often inflicted on the victim whether this was with a shovel, hammer, knife, or by gunshot.[3,4,12,13,15,19,21] Reports of aggressive events being repeated on different nights were rare.[1,12]

Sensory Perception

There was little documentation about the sensory perception of the aggressor, probably in part because of the often fatal outcome for the witness. The subject's eyes were recorded as being open in one individual,[1] but in this and all the other reports there seems to have been a failure to recognize the identity of the victim. There was a lack of response to the noise of a gunshot during the episode[3] and no response to pain from a severe self-inflicted injury.[3]

Emotional Expression

The only comment about emotional expression during the sleep violence was one report of an appearance of satisfaction while sleepwalking after attacking the victim.[11] In none of the events was there any suggestion that the aggressor expressed any fear or anger during the violent act itself. However, a feeling of horror or fear on waking after the event was recognized.[3,6,11] Two subjects subsequently attempted suicide because of what they had done.[3,13]

Dream Recall

In several reports there were perceptions of being attacked or surrounded by ghosts,[7] evil spirits,[3] fire,[2] wild beasts,[1] shadowy figures,[12] burglars,[7] soldiers,[12] or other strangers,[3,12] or of being seized by the hair.[21] In the fatal self-violent episode the subject felt that he was surrounded by enemies and an evil spirit told him to kill himself.[3] One individual dreamt of murdering the person who he subsequently tried to attack.[11]

Recall of Events

A lack of recall of the events was a feature of these reports. Two subjects were aware that they had shot someone, but were uncertain who,[8,22] and another had difficulty understanding how the violence had been carried out.[1]

Trigger Factors

Several of the events were triggered by physical stimulation of the subject immediately before-hand[2,7,8,16,21-23] or by loud noises.[2] In others there had been similar physical activity during the day, such as for the subject who was chopping wood and then killed his bed partner with an axe at night.[12] In several reports there had been psychological stress immediately before the event, such as a quarrel,[18] a threatened attack,[5,22] or argument,[15] but in two cases the stress had been more long-standing.[2,7] Sleep deprivation was mentioned in only one report.[21] Several of the subjects had previously been sleepwalkers.[5,8,22,23]

Premeditation

In no case was there any evidence for any premeditation of the attack, or any motive. One subject raised the alarm about the episode afterwards.[5]

DISCUSSION

Sleep violence has been the subject of several reviews and case reports over the last 25 years.[14,24-35] These reports have elucidated many aspects of sleep violence, but the detailed characteristics of the violence itself and the behavior of the aggressor are poorly documented both in these reports and in current textbooks on sleep medicine.

The case histories in this review almost certainly represent the extreme of sleep violence. These episodes were more likely to arouse public attention and to result in criminal arrest. For the same reasons, however, it is less likely that many episodes went unreported, particularly once the legal community, in the wake of a growing medical interest, became increasingly aware of sleep violence during the nineteenth century.

Among early physicians, a consensus of opinion stressed the unconscious nature of sleep violence. Not unlike the behavior of sleepwalkers, violence under such circumstances was involuntary. While acknowledging that diagnoses could

be problematic in the eyes of the law, French physicians,[36,37] in adopting this belief, were shortly followed by medical authorities on both sides of the Atlantic.[20] In *The Medical Jurisprudence of Insanity*,[38] the well-known English psychiatrist John MacMichan Pagan drew attention as well to violence arising from victims' night terrors or their abrupt arousal from a state of sleep.

Sleep violence can be a manifestation of REM sleep behavior disorder, particularly in older subjects,[39] obstructive sleep apneas,[40] epilepsy,[41] narcolepsy,[42,43] posttraumatic stress disorder, and psychogenic dissociative disorders (**Table 1**).[44] It should also be distinguished from violence carried out at night while the subject is awake, even when this is subsequently denied.[12,17,45] In this series patients with features characteristic of these various disorders were excluded. The REM sleep behavior disorder may also have been less frequent in the past because fewer males lived beyond the age of 55 years, and obstructive sleep apneas may also have been less common because of the relative rarity of obesity at the time of these reports.

In most cases sleep violence is caused by an arousal disorder from non-REM sleep, usually stages 3 and 4, but there is a dissociation of the sleep-wake state between different parts of the brain so that areas such as the motor and cingulate cortex function as in wakefulness whereas association areas, particularly the frontal cortex, function as in sleep.[46,47] Defensive and aggressive behaviors are thought to be initiated particularly in the orbitomedial region of the frontal lobes,[48,49] but also in the medial hypothalamus and amygdala.[50] Damage to these areas may lead to aggressive behavior.[51] In arousal disorders characterized by sleep violence, presumably one or more of these areas is activated in addition to those that contribute to nonviolent sleep terrors.

Most of these subjects with sleep violence due to arousal disorders were young and male. A previous history of sleepwalking was often recognized. In some, stress over a few days before the event, but more particularly on the day before

Table 1 Causes of sleep violence	
Non-REM sleep disorders	Arousal disorders Posttraumatic stress disorder Obstructive sleep apneas Epilepsy
REM sleep disorders	REM sleep behavior disorder Status dissociatus Narcolepsy

the violence, may have triggered the episode. In several it was provoked by physical stimulation of the sleeper, which presumably caused a partial arousal from sleep.[52,53]

In some individuals[7,54] the sleep violence appeared to form part of a confusional arousal at the end of an episode of sleepwalking. Contact or restraint by another person appeared to convert a nonviolent sleepwalking episode into a violent confusional arousal. This finding would explain how some of the episodes of sleep violence occurred at a distance from the patient's bed. However, as was recognized in a previous review,[52] none of the subjects had in any premeditated way sought out the victim.

A characteristic of these reports was that the attack often involved repetitive movements, for instance, repeated stabbing or shooting. These relatively simple and stereotyped behaviors may have been the result of activation of central pattern generators in the spinal cord and brain stem,[55,56] which are responsible for innate rather than reflex behavioral patterns such as walking and swimming. These behaviors are normally inhibited by higher centers, particularly in the cerebral cortex and basal ganglia, but in sleep violence they may be released from this control. Some of the attacks, however, required learned activities such as shooting, which presumably involved activation of cortical motor and executive areas as well.

In several reports the aggressor was noted to have failed to recognize the victim despite his eyes being open. This finding suggests that although visual perception and spatial awareness were sufficient to enable the individual to direct violence effectively and precisely, the higher visual interpretative centers responsible for facial recognition, particularly in the fusiform gyrus, were inactive. A lack of awareness of other aspects of the environment, such as noise, as well as pain felt by the aggressor was frequently documented.

The interpretation of dreamlike mentation is difficult retrospectively, because these recollections can range from complex narratives through to recall of simple images, such as of animals or people attacking or chasing the subject, or just a more general sensation of fear or impending death. The latter, which is a feature of sleep terrors, was reported for several episodes whereby the subject acted violently with the intent of protecting a member of the family, but misinterpreted the situation so that it was a family member or bed partner who was inadvertently attacked.

The absence of any recall of the aggressive events suggests that some of the higher cortical association centers, possibly related to the hippocampus and medial temporal lobe, were inactive at the time of the attack. Some subjects, however, were aware of a sensation of fear or horror immediately after the event as well as being able to recall the content of dreamlike events as they returned to a normal level of awareness.

The limitations of this study are that the cases were not reported systematically, the degree of detail varied between case reports, the events occurred over a long time period, and none of the subjects underwent objective physiologic testing as would be standard practice in modern sleep medicine departments. Nevertheless, the pattern of clinical features in each case suggested that the events were attributable to an arousal disorder.

The case histories in this review probably represent the extremes of sleep violence, and therefore in many ways are able to provide clear indications about the nature of these events. The descriptions suggest remarkable consistency in the phenotype of arousal disorders leading to sleep violence during the last 500 years, although demographic factors, such as the age and obesity of the population, may have influenced the prevalence of other causes of sleep violence. The combination of aggression, lack of facial recognition, and lack of recall of the episodes documented in this extensive series characterize sleep violence caused by an arousal disorder. Presumably this requires not only activation of central neural mechanisms leading to intense emotion, often fear, but also of specific centers, probably in the frontal cortex, hypothalamus, and amygdala, which enable this to be expressed as aggressive behavior during sleep.

REFERENCES

1. Yellowlees D. Homicide by a somnambulist. J Mental Sci 1878;24:451–8.
2. Bonkalo A. Impulsive acts and confusional states during incomplete arousal from sleep: criminological and forensic implications. Psychiatr Q 1974;48:400–9.
3. Poldosky E. Somnambulistic homicide. Dis Nerv Syst 1959;20:534–6.
4. Beieri A. Tractatio Juridica de Jure Dormientium. Magdeburg (Germany): Aere Hendeliano; 1726.
5. National Police Gazette. Killed in his sleep. National Police Gazette vol. 36, August 21, 1880. p. 152.
6. The history of man. Religion and philosophy, vol. 2. London: M. Cooper; 1746. p. 160–72. Chapter LXXV of Sleep Walkers; etc.
7. Gudden H. Die physiologische und pathologische Schlaf-trunkenheit. Archiv fur Psychiatrie Nervenkrankheiten 1905;40:989–1015 [in German].

8. Kentucky Court of Appeals. Central Law Journal January 23 1880;10:4.

9. Wanley N. The wonders of the little world etc. London: T. Davies; 1774. p. 624–9.

10. Murder will out. National Police Gazette 41, November 25, 1882.

11. Somnambulism. The North American Miscellany; A weekly magazine of choice selections. June 21, 1851;2:21.

12. Howard C, D'Orban PT. Violence in sleep: medicolegal issues and two case reports. Psychol Med 1987;17:915–25.

13. Hopwood JS, Snell HK. Amnesia in relation to crime. Journal of Mental Science 1933;79:27–41.

14. Oswald I, Evans J. On serious violence during sleep-walking. Br J Psychiatry 1985;147:688–91.

15. Hill D, Sargant W. A case of matricide. Lancet 1943; 241:526–7.

16. Somnambulism. In: The Family Economist, vol. 1. London; 1857. p. 78.

17. Natural somnambulism. Boston Med Surg J 1846; 34:10.

18. Joubert L. Treatise on laughter. Tuscaloosa (AL): University of Alabama Press; 1980.

19. Proceedings of the Old Bailey. 1674–1913. June 13, 1853.

20. Walker N. Crime and insanity in England, vol. 1, the historical perspective. Edinburgh (United Kingdom): Edinburgh University Press; 1968. p. 166–9.

21. Buchner in Henke's Journal of Medical Jurisprudence. Melbourne, 1870.

22. Court of Appeals of Kentucky. Fain v The Commonwealth. November 18, 1879.

23. Kentucky Court of Appeals, Fain v the Commonwealth. Central Law Journal, January 23, 1880;10:4.

24. Morissettte L. Homicidal somnambulism. Sleep 1995;18:805.

25. Moldofsky H, Gilbert R, Lue FA, et al. Sleep-related violence. Sleep 1995;18:731–9.

26. Broughton RJ, Shimizu T. Sleep-related violence: a medical and forensic challenge. Sleep 1995;18:727–30.

27. Thomas TN. Sleepwalking disorder and mens rea: a review and case report. J Forensic Sci 1997;42: 17–24.

28. Ohayon MM, Caulet M, Priest RG. Violent behavior during sleep. J Clin Psychiatry 1997;58:369–76.

29. Mahowald MW, Schenck CH. Complex motor behavior arising during the sleep period: forensic science implications. Sleep 1995;18:724–7.

30. Guilleminault C, Moscovitch A, Leger D. Injury, violence and nocturnal wanderings. Am J Forensic Psych 1995;16:33–46.

31. Gilmore JV. Murdering while asleep: clinical and forensic issues. Forensic Rep 1991;4:455–9.

32. Guilleminault C, Leger D, Philip P, et al. Nocturnal wandering and violence: review of a sleep clinic population. J Forensic Sci 1998;43:158–63.

33. Ovuga EB. Murder during sleep-walking. East Afr Med J 1992;69:533–4.

34. Guilleminault C, Moscovitch A, Leger D. Forensic sleep medicine: nocturnal wandering and violence. Sleep 1995;18:740–8.

35. Shneerson JM. Sleep violence. Br J Hosp Med 2009; 70:332–5.

36. Georget ET. Examen medical des proces criminels. Paris: Migneret; 1825. p. 116 [in French].

37. Marc CC. De la folie: considere dans ses rapports avec les questions medico-judiciaires, vol. 2. Paris: J-B Bailliere; 1840. p. 668 [in French].

38. Pagan JM. The medical jurisprudence of insanity. London: Ball Arnold & Co; 1840. p. 325–7.

39. Chambers's information for the people. An account of a human body. London: Orr and Smith; 1835. p. 61–2.

40. Nofzinger EA, Wettstein RM. Homicidal behavior and sleep apnea: a case report and medicolegal discussion. Sleep 1995;18:776–82.

41. Borum R, Appelbaum KL. Epilepsy, aggression, and criminal responsibility. Psychiatr Serv 1996;47:762–3.

42. Szucs A, Janszky J, Hollo A, et al. Misleading hallucinations in unrecognized narcolepsy. Acta Psychiatr Scand 2003;108:314–7.

43. Zorick FJ, Salis PJ, Roth T, et al. Narcolepsy and automatic behavior: a case report. J Clin Psychiatry 1979;40:194–7.

44. Agargun MY, Kara H, Ozer OA, et al. Sleep-related violence, dissociative experiences, and childhood traumatic events. Sleep Hypn 2002;4:52–7.

45. Murder trials and executions in New Hampshire. Report of the trial of Abraham Prescott for the murder of Mrs Sally Cochran, of Pembroke, June 23 1833. Manchester (NH): Daily Mirror Office; 1869.

46. Bassetti C, Vella S, Donati F, et al. SPECT during sleepwalking. Lancet 2000;356:484–5.

47. Terzaghi M, Sartori I, Tassi L, et al. Evidence of dissociated arousal states during NREM Parasomnia from an intracerebral neurophysiological study. Sleep 2009;32:409–12.

48. Grafman J, Schwab K, Warden D, et al. Frontal lobe injuries, violence, and aggressions: a report of the Vietnam Head Injury Study. Neurology 1996;46:1231–8.

49. Brower MC, Price BH. Neuropsychiatry of frontal lobe dysfunction in violent and criminal behaviour: a critical review. J Neurol Neurosurg Psychiatry 2001;71:720–6.

50. Albert DJ, Walsh ML, Jonik RH. Aggression in humans: what is its biological foundation? Neurosci Biobehav Rev 1993;17:405–25.

51. Hawkins KA, Trobst KK. Frontal lobe dysfunction and aggression: conceptual issues and research findings. Agg Violent Behav 2000;5:147–57.

52. Pressman MR. Disorders of arousal from sleep and violent behavior: the role of physical contact and proximity. Sleep 2007;30:1039–47.

53. Pressman MR. Factors that predispose, prime and precipitate NREM parasomnias in adults: clinical and forensic implications. Sleep Med Rev 2007;11: 5–30.

54. Schmidt G. Die Verbrechen in der Schlaftrunkenheit. Zeitschrift fur die Gesamte Neurologie und Psychiatrie 1943;176:208–54 [in German].

55. Tassinari CA, Rubboli G, Gaardella E, et al. Central pattern generators for a common semiology in fronto-limbic seizures and in parasomnias. A neuro-ethologic approach. Neurol Sci 2005;26:s225–32.

56. Marder E, Bucher D. Central pattern generators and the control of rhythmic movements. Curr Biol 2001; 11:R986–96.

Index

United States Postal Service

Statement of Ownership, Management, and Circulation
(All Periodicals Publications Except Requestor Publications)

1. Publication Title

Sleep Medicine Clinics of North America

2. Publication Number

0 2 5 - 0 5 3

3. Filing Date

9/16/11

4. Issue Frequency

Mar, Jun, Sep, Dec

5. Number of Issues Published Annually

4

6. Annual Subscription Price

$161.00

7. Complete Mailing Address of Known Office of Publication *(Not printer) (Street, city, county, state, and ZIP+4®)*

Elsevier Inc.
360 Park Avenue South
New York, NY 10010-1710

Contact Person

Amy S. Beacham

Telephone *(Include area code)*

215-239-3687

8. Complete Mailing Address of Headquarters or General Business Office of Publisher *(Not printer)*

Elsevier Inc., 360 Park Avenue South, New York, NY 10010-1710

9. Full Names and Complete Mailing Addresses of Publisher, Editor, and Managing Editor *(Do not leave blank)*

Publisher *(Name and complete mailing address)*

Kim Murphy, Elsevier, Inc., 1600 John F. Kennedy Blvd. Suite 1800, Philadelphia, PA 19103-2899

Editor *(Name and complete mailing address)*

Sarah Barth, Elsevier, Inc., 1600 John F. Kennedy Blvd. Suite 1800, Philadelphia, PA 19103-2899

Managing Editor *(Name and complete mailing address)*

Sarah Barth, Elsevier, Inc., 1600 John F. Kennedy Blvd. Suite 1800, Philadelphia, PA 19103-2899

10. Owner *(Do not leave blank. If the publication is owned by a corporation, give the name and address of the corporation immediately followed by the names and addresses of all stockholders owning or holding 1 percent or more of the total amount of stock. If not owned by a corporation, give the names and addresses of the individual owners. If owned by a partnership or other unincorporated firm, give its name and address as well as those of each individual owner. If the publication is published by a nonprofit organization, give its name and address.)*

Full Name	Complete Mailing Address
Wholly owned subsidiary of	4520 East-West Highway
Reed/Elsevier, US holdings	Bethesda, MD 20814

11. Known Bondholders, Mortgagees, and Other Security Holders Owning or Holding 1 Percent or More of Total Amount of Bonds, Mortgages, or Other Securities. If none, check box. ☐ None

Full Name	Complete Mailing Address
N/A	

12. Tax Status *(For completion by nonprofit organizations authorized to mail at nonprofit rates) (Check one)*

The purpose, function, and nonprofit status of this organization and the exempt status for federal income tax purposes:

☐ Has Not Changed During Preceding 12 Months
☐ Has Changed During Preceding 12 Months *(Publisher must submit explanation of change with this statement)*

PS Form 3526, September 2007 (Page 1 of 3 (Instructions Page 3)) PSN 7530-01-000-9931 PRIVACY NOTICE: See our Privacy policy in www.usps.com

---

13. Publication Title

Sleep Medicine Clinics of North America

14. Issue Date for Circulation Data Below

September 2011

15. Extent and Nature of Circulation

			Average No. Copies Each Issue During Preceding 12 Months	No. Copies of Single Issue Published Nearest to Filing Date
a. Total Number of Copies *(Net press run)*			918	690
b. Paid Circulation (By Mail and Outside the Mail)	(1)	Mailed Outside-County Paid Subscriptions Stated on PS Form 3541. *(Include paid distribution above nominal rate, advertiser's proof copies, and exchange copies)*	486	461
	(2)	Mailed In-County Paid Subscriptions Stated on PS Form 3541 *(Include paid distribution above nominal rate, advertiser's proof copies, and exchange copies)*		
	(3)	Paid Distribution Outside the Mails Including Sales Through Dealers and Carriers, Street Vendors, Counter Sales, and Other Paid Distribution Outside USPS®	39	34
	(4)	Paid Distribution by Other Classes Mailed Through the USPS (e.g. First-Class Mail®)		
c. Total Paid Distribution *(Sum of 15b (1), (2), (3), and (4))*		►	525	495
d. Free or Nominal Rate Distribution (By Mail and Outside the Mail)	(1)	Free or Nominal Rate Outside-County Copies Included on PS Form 3541	57	53
	(2)	Free or Nominal Rate In-County Copies Included on PS Form 3541		
	(3)	Free or Nominal Rate Copies Mailed at Other Classes Through the USPS (e.g. First-Class Mail)		
	(4)	Free or Nominal Rate Distribution Outside the Mail (Carriers or other means)		
e. Total Free or Nominal Rate Distribution *(Sum of 15d (1), (2), (3) and (4))*		►	57	53
f. Total Distribution *(Sum of 15c and 15e)*		►	582	548
g. Copies not Distributed *(See instructions to publishers #4 (page #3))*		►	336	142
h. Total *(Sum of 15f and g)*		►	918	690
i. Percent Paid *(15c divided by 15f times 100)*		►	90.21%	90.33%

16. Publication of Statement of Ownership

☐ If the publication is a general publication, publication of this statement is required. Will be printed in the **December 2011** issue of this publication. ☐ Publication not required

17. Signature and Title of Editor, Publisher, Business Manager, or Owner

[signature] Amy S. Beacham – Senior Inventory Distribution Coordinator

Date

September 16, 2011

I certify that all information furnished on this form is true and complete. I understand that anyone who furnishes false or misleading information on this form or who omits material or information requested on the form may be subject to criminal sanctions (including fines and imprisonment) and/or civil sanctions (including civil penalties).

PS Form 3526, September 2007 (Page 2 of 3)